BUILDING HEALTH, BUILDING WELLNESS

To Jim & Gail:

Best of Health!

To Jim Still,

Best Wishes!

[signature]

BUILDING HEALTH, BUILDING WELLNESS

A COMMONSENSE APPROACH TO HEALTH ENHANCEMENT

GREGORY W. PIERCE, MD

iUniverse, Inc.
Bloomington

BUILDING HEALTH, BUILDING WELLNESS
A COMMONSENSE APPROACH TO HEALTH ENHANCEMENT

Copyright © 2012 by Gregory W. Pierce, MD.

All rights reserved. No part of this book may be used or reproduced by any means, graphic, electronic, or mechanical, including photocopying, recording, taping or by any information storage retrieval system without the written permission of the publisher except in the case of brief quotations embodied in critical articles and reviews.

You should not undertake any diet/exercise regimen recommended in this book before consulting your personal physician. Neither the author nor the publisher shall be responsible or liable for any loss or damage allegedly arising as a consequence of your use or application of any information or suggestions contained in this book.

The information presented in this book is true and complete to the best of the knowledge of the author and publisher. This book is intended for information only and should not be used to replace, countermand, or conflict with the advice given to readers by their personal physician. It is not a substitute for examination, diagnosis, and medical care provided by a licensed and qualified health professional. Readers are advised to consult their personal physician before undertaking any changes in their health or wellness care. The author and publisher disclaim all liability in connection with the specific personal use of any and all information provided in this book by any person.

iUniverse books may be ordered through booksellers or by contacting:

iUniverse
1663 Liberty Drive
Bloomington, IN 47403
www.iuniverse.com
1-800-Authors (1-800-288-4677)

Because of the dynamic nature of the Internet, any web addresses or links contained in this book may have changed since publication and may no longer be valid. The views expressed in this work are solely those of the author and do not necessarily reflect the views of the publisher, and the publisher hereby disclaims any responsibility for them.

Any people depicted in stock imagery provided by Thinkstock are models, and such images are being used for illustrative purposes only.
Certain stock imagery © Thinkstock.

ISBN: 978-1-4697-8754-1 (sc)
ISBN: 978-1-4697-8755-8 (ebk)

Printed in the United States of America

iUniverse rev. date: 04/27/2012

For Raymond and Ollie Pierce, Kannie and Essie Mae Brundidge, Raymond and Geraldine Pierce, and all of the "Giants" upon whose shoulders I stand; Eurica, the Giant at my side, and Matthew and Gregory, the Giants on the way.

Therefore everyone who hears these words of mine and puts them into practice is like a wise man who built his house on the rock. The rain came down, the streams rose, and the winds blew and beat against that house; yet it did not fall, because it had its foundation on the rock. But everyone who hears these words of mine and does not put them into practice is like a foolish man who built his house on sand. The rain came down, the streams rose, and the winds blew and beat against that house, and it fell with a great crash.
—Matthew 7:24-27

Men do not stumble over mountains, but over molehills.
—Confucius

Contents

Foreword xi

Preface xiii

Acknowledgments xvii

Part I — **The Physical Self** 1
    Introduction: Why Do Diets Fail? 3
    Chapter 1 — Weight Loss: Goal or Guide? 7
    Chapter 2 — Nutrients 12
    Chapter 3 — Activity 27
    Chapter 4 — Stress 33
    Chapter 5 — Environmental Factors 36

Part II — **Beyond the Physical** 43
    Chapter 6 — The Family & Community 45
    Chapter 7 — The Inner Self 48

Part III — **Putting It All Together** 55
    Chapter 8 — The PIERCE RECIPE 57
    Chapter 9 — Getting Started 63
    Chapter 10 — Do You! 68
    Chapter 11 — Fine Tuning: Turning Failure into Success 70
    Conclusion: A Life of Greatness 73

Foreword

This foreword is dedicated to my friend and colleague, Dr. Gregory Pierce, who single-handedly restored my faith in the purity, generosity, and humanity that exist in the medical profession. The importance and enormity of his writings will forever alter the philosophical landscape of America and the world. His clarity of vision, intensity of purpose, endless dedication, craftsmanship, and joy have given life to this book. I thank him for teaching us how to ask questions of our physicians, look to the heavens for inspiration, and listen to our bodies for the Truth.

In his marvelous book *Building Health, Building Wellness*, Dr. Gregory Pierce talks about how potential setbacks in health can lead to strong comebacks in overall wellness.

How apropos it is that Dr. Pierce concludes his book with a discussion of "A Life of Greatness." In person, he frequently responds to the greeting "How are you?" with "Life is good!" This book is just one example of how Dr. Pierce constantly inspires with his courage and generosity. Recently when I was asked in an interview about any reads, people, or events that served as a pivotal or "aha" moment in my life, I pondered only a few seconds. I believe life is a continual learning process, so it was a challenge for me to single out one specific turning point when something I read or someone I met made all the difference, but I am inspired constantly by the writings of Dr. Pierce. His appetite for life comes through in his wellness seminars, and his *joie de vivre* is contagious for everyone around him.

The PIERCE Recipe will indeed work if you apply it to your life. In life, we have to deal with the part of us that says, "I can't do it." We have to rely on the part of us that says, "Run your own race, baby!" We sometimes must ask ourselves whether we are running our race or someone else's. Whether or not we know it, individuals carry their own unique slogan or saying that resonates throughout their lives. This commonsense approach to health enhancement makes sense! Now is the time to "turn your stumbling blocks into building blocks." Remember—in life, it is the things that you do not do that you regret, not the things that you do.

Today is the first day of your new life.

Adolph Brown, III, PsyD

Dr. Brown is a Master Teacher, psychologist, and author of Real Talk: Lessons in Uncommon Sense *and* Championship Habits: Soft Skills in Hard Times for Leaders and Managers.

Preface

"But, Dr. Pierce, I do exercise, and I don't eat that much. I just don't understand why it is so hard for me to lose weight!" After a dozen years as a family physician, I had heard this said in some form many times before. Everyone seems to overestimate what they are doing and underestimate what it takes to make real changes, and it is up to me to be the bad guy and tell them the truth. However, that day I had a different thought: *What if this lady isn't lying to me, and what if she isn't crazy? I have heard this story so many times before; could they all be lying? Could they all be crazy?*

I started my medical life as a traditional family doctor. As the third doctor in the group that I joined in a semirural town in Tennessee, we did it all. In addition to our office practice, we delivered babies, took care of patients in the hospital and nursing homes, and even made house calls from time to time. Not quite a *Marcus Welby, MD* lifestyle, but close.

Six years later, marriage and a move to a more urban location in Virginia led me to a practice in an urgent care center. Sprained ankles and sore throats were staples of my day. Management of ongoing problems such as diabetes and hypertension were a thing of the past—almost. As the medical environment changed, we increasingly became more involved in providing ongoing care to our patients. Having been away from this style of practice for a while, I came back to it with a new perspective. I saw the same types of patients with the same types of problems; however, I noticed things that I had not noticed in the past.

For example, at the end of a clinical encounter, a patient said, "Oh, by the way, Dr. Pierce, could you check my B_{12} level?"

Only having seen her for an urgent care problem, I didn't have an extensive medical history for her. "Why would you need to know that?" I asked.

"Well, when they did my gastric bypass surgery several years ago, they told me to keep an eye on it."

I wondered, *As overweight as she is, how could she have had surgery for weight loss?* As time went on, I encountered several others who had had similar surgery but continued to be "overweight."

This got me to thinking about weight loss in general. If surgery fails, what about other methods? I really hadn't given it much thought before, but I began to notice that they *all* seemed to fail. It seemed that every advertisement for a diet or exercise program had its successes proudly displayed with a disclaimer that read, "Results not typical." If these good results are not typical, what are the typical results? Most plans had good short-term results, but long-term results were modest at best. Perhaps that is why there are so many methods—not because they all work, but because they all fail! If one method worked for everyone all of the time, that method would be the only one needed.

The next question is, "*Why* do they all fail?" After much thought and research, I came to the conclusion that the reason diet and exercise programs fail is not that they are not good, but that they are not the right *program* for the right *person* at the right *time*.

This sounds simple but actually speaks to the marked complexity that is the human body and the human social condition. Too often we think of health and wellness only in physical terms. Diet and exercise are only part of the equation that describes what it takes to attain and maintain optimal health and well-being. To fully understand ourselves and each other, we must also attempt to understand our environment, including family and community factors, and those factors that make us tick: our sense of self-awareness (mental/psychology) and our sense of our place in the world or universe (spirituality).

Envision a "Table of Wellness" with four legs representing the major aspects of our lives that determine our sense of wellness: the Physical, Mental, Social, and Spiritual. If one or more of these legs is short (weak or underdeveloped), the entire table leans, rocks, or is otherwise unstable. Complete wellness means paying attention to all of these factors.

This book is my attempt to help you, the average person, to tease through the massive amounts of information available in print and online to try to make sense of what is available and to determine what the best approach is for you at this time to improve your health.

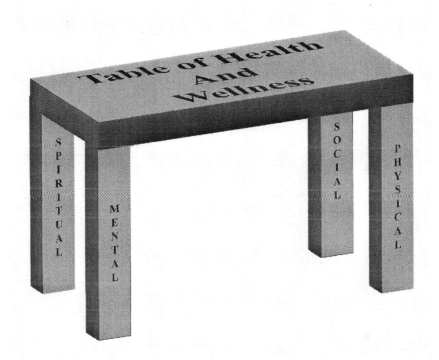

Acknowledgments

Many thanks to all of those involved in the production of this work, including all of those who have had a hand in teaching me all along the way, including my parents, teachers, and colleagues, as well as my patients, who continue to educate me.

Thanks to Dr. Adolph Brown, Mrs. Marla Brown, Mrs. Jodi Stambaugh, and Dr. Eurica Hill for invaluable advice and review of this book.

A final thanks to my wife, Eurica, and my sons, Gregory and Matthew, for their continued love and support.

PART I

THE PHYSICAL SELF

INTRODUCTION

Why Do Diets Fail?

We hear the news every day. We Americans are overweight. Obesity is an epidemic. Chronic diseases are killing us at escalating rates. The main reason (we are told) that we are so unhealthy is that we are lazy and gluttonous. All we need do is exercise more and eat less, and we will be successful in achieving perfect health.

Despite this simple prescription, we are not perfectly healthy. This is despite living in a country in which we spend billions of dollars each year on "solutions" like diet and exercise books, diet and exercise clinics, diet and exercise videos, diet and exercise websites, diet and exercise supplements, diet and exercise equipment, diet and exercise programs, and diet and exercise professionals. Heavily advertised and endorsed by well-qualified, well-meaning experts and users, each program proudly shows its successful customers, often followed by that familiar disclaimer: "Results may not be typical."

Why is it that we have not been able to buy our way into better health? Why is it that we seem to be failing as a nation? Why is it that so many of us seem to fail more often than we succeed?

The next time that you are at the mall, try this experiment. Look at peoples' feet. Keep looking until you find someone wearing the exact same style, color, and size shoe that you are wearing. Keep track of how many feet you have to look at until you find shoes that exactly match yours. How many different types and sizes of shoe did you see? Why is it that we need so many different types, styles, and sizes of shoe? Are our feet really that different? Now, think of how different we are physically, physiologically, biochemically, culturally, and genetically. Given these differences, is it reasonable to expect that we all would need or benefit from the same diet and activity program?

Now consider how many shoes you own. Why do you have more than one pair? You only have one pair of feet! It's obvious that you need and like to have different types of shoes for different occasions and purposes. Think of how many factors go into deciding what type of shoe to wear. What will you be doing? What is the weather like? What styles do you like or not like? What type of shoe is available where you shop? What type of shoe can you afford? What clothes will you wear with the shoes? Sometimes, the exact shoe that you want is not available in your size, so you have to compromise.

Think of how many shoes that you have worn in your life. It is obvious that you and your feet change over time. The same size that you wore five years ago may not fit now. You may now like a newer style of shoe. Is it reasonable to expect, then, that your dietary and activity needs would be the same from day to day for your entire life?

How does this compare with what we have experienced when trying to improve our health with a formal diet or exercise program? We find that many of them are "one size fits all" (everyone should wear a size 10D); many are too narrow in focus (all you need are loafers); and many don't consider our individuality and uniqueness (even if you don't like burgundy wingtips and have flat feet, this shoe will work for you if you wear it right). Somewhere along the line, we learn how to buy shoes that are comfortable and functional for us. There are people and tools available to help us to sort through all of the shoes that are available and find the right pair with the right fit that suits our taste. Perhaps we need a way to sort through all of the health information that is available in order to find the right style and "fit" for each of us.

In this book, we will review a variety of approaches and explore why they may or may not be appropriate for an individual, along with strategies for implementing changes. We will discuss the many factors that actually determine our overall health and well-being, beyond diet and exercise.

The goal is to help us to turn what may have previously been "stumbling blocks" into "building blocks" and turn our failures into success. Consider this as a guiding principle as you read this book: Success is doing what is best for me at this time, realizing that what I need to do will change as I change. It is the process of constant improvement that is important, not just reaching specific goals. Optimal health is a journey of living, not a specific destination.

Let's get ready to be successful!

The Basics

Let us start by defining a few terms that will be used in this book. (Don't get intimidated by the terminology. You can skip this part and return to it later if you have questions about a word.)

What is a calorie?

The scientific definition of a calorie is "the amount of heat required at a pressure of one atmosphere to raise the temperature of one gram (about 1/28 of an ounce) of water one degree Celcius."[1] When it comes to food, it is the amount of food that it would take to produce this same amount of heat (energy). Different types of foods produce different amounts of calories. Carbohydrates and proteins produce 4 calories per gram, and fat 9 calories per gram. Alcohol produces 7 calories per gram, but has no nutritive value.

So the next time that you read a food label and it says that one serving of cashews has 160 calories, it means that if you digested and metabolized the cashews, the amount of energy produced would be 160 calories. It is assumed that this is the amount of energy that will be transferred to you when you eat the cashews.

It is estimated that the average man needs to consume 24 calories every day for every kilogram (about 2.2 pounds) that he weighs. For the average woman, the number is 22 calories. But remember, this book is not about what is average. It is about you.

What are carbohydrates?

Although a misnomer, the name refers to the fact that chemically, these compounds contain the molecules of carbon (carbo-) and water (hydrate). These are the sugars, starches, and fiber that we eat.

What are fats?

Fat refers to the soft, greasy material that is found in animals and plants. You may also see the terms "fatty acids" or "lipids" used when referring to this category of food. Although we tend to think of fat as

---

[1] Merriam-Webster Online Dictionary copyright © 2012 by Merriam-Webster, Incorporated

being bad when it comes to food, we will see how necessary and desirable certain fats are for our health.

What are proteins?
The word comes from the Greek word "protos" which means "first." This refers to the fact that proteins are the major component of animals and plants. Proteins are made of small chemical building blocks called amino acids. Our bodies can make some of these amino acids, but not others. Therefore, we are dependent on our diet to make sure that we have all of the amino acids necessary to make proteins, which are used to make structures such as muscle.

What are vitamins?
Derived from the word "vita," which means "life", it was thought at one time that all of these substances contained amino acids, "amines." Even though this original idea is now known not to be true, these compounds are nonetheless "vital" for the normal growth and functioning of our bodies.

What are minerals?
From the Latin word for "mine," these are substances found in the crust of the earth. There are several minerals that are necessary for our health, and there are others that can be detrimental to our health.

What is a cell?
Cells are the basic units of structure for our bodies. Each cell contains a nucleus that holds genetic material, or genes.

What are genes?
From the Greek word "genos," which means "birth," these are the chemical units that carry all of the information that each cell of our body needs to operate. Often referred to as a "blueprint," genes tell the cells how to put together amino acids in order to make certain proteins. The proteins then do the work of the cell.

What is nutrition?
From the Latin word meaning "to nurse" or "to nourish," this word refers to the quality of the food that we eat. As you probably suspect, not all food is equally nourishing.

CHAPTER 1

WEIGHT LOSS: GOAL OR GUIDE?

Stumbling Block #1: "I'm overweight" or "I must go on a diet in order to be healthy."

Is weight loss a goal to be achieved or a process that we go through on the way to better health? Without a doubt, we are an image-oriented society—what you see is what you get. When it comes to our personal image, weight is perceived to be of paramount importance. We are bombarded with messages of the unhealthy effects of obesity and how overweight individuals are at risk for many health problems and, ultimately, early death.

We traditionally equate being "overweight" with being "obese" and with being "fat." That last term seems to ring the truest for most of us. While it may be partially true, perhaps a more in-depth look will give us a different perception.

BMI: The Body Mass Index is a calculation based on weight and height. (BMI=weight (kg) / [height (m)]^2 or weight (lb) / [height (in)]^2 x 703). The resulting number is used to define ranges of weight, with less than 18.5 being considered underweight; 18.5–24.9 normal weight; 25.0–29.9 overweight; and above 30.0 considered obese. This might be useful as a starting point, but built into this number is an assumption that everyone of a certain height has the same amount of "non-fat" weight. That is, the only reason that one's BMI could vary is due to the amount of fat that is present. Proponents of this concept readily admit that the BMI is not accurate for those who are very young, very old, or very muscular. Why not? People in these groups are known to have differences in muscle mass that confounds the calculation of the BMI. Then why use BMI as a parameter of health? It is convenient and accurate for many people, but does it really tell us all that we need to know?

Our weight or mass is composed of several things: muscle, fat and everything else, like bone and water (including blood and other liquids in the body). This category is probably the most consistent from person to person at a given stature, while the fat and muscle mass are probably the most variable. Because the BMI does not take into account differences in muscle mass, it may not be the most accurate indication of health.

Waist-Hip Ratio: The waist-hip ratio (WHR) is obtained by dividing the measurement around the body at the waist (at or just above the level of the belly button) by the measurement around the body at the widest part of the hips or buttocks. Some like to use this as a measure of health and the risk of disease because it considers differences in body structure. The ideal ratio for men is considered to be about 0.9 and for women about 0.7. Ratios above these indicate more fat in the abdomen than the hips ("apple shaped") and are associated with more health problems than lower ratios ("pear shape"), in which there is more fat at the hips.

The waist measurement itself can also be used as a rough guide to health. In general, most men begin to experience an increased risk for health problems when the waist size is greater than 37 inches, with the ideal being less than 35 inches. In women, the risk goes up at about 32 inches, with ideal being less than 30 inches.

Body Composition: The concept of body composition may be more useful when it comes to thinking about our health. A weight of 200 pounds doesn't tell us much unless we know what makes up those 200 pounds. Two hundred pounds with 28 percent fat is certainly different from 200 pounds with 16 percent fat. Body builders are well aware of this and are noted to have a body mass index that might put them in the obese range, although they might have a very low percentage of body fat. True, these individuals are more the exception than the rule, but it changes our perspective when we stop thinking just about total weight loss as a goal and start to think about losing unnecessary fat and building or maintaining muscle mass. This is an important distinction. The amount of fat that we carry can be measured or estimated in several ways, including the use electronic handheld devices, electronic scales, and calipers. The most accurate measurement of body fat is obtained by taking measurements floating in a tank of water, which is not practical for most of us!

Is Weight Loss Healthy? Is fat, in and of itself, necessarily a bad thing? After all, it does exist for a reason, and it may be more than just a passive repository for energy. Fat actually performs useful functions and only represents a problem when certain types of body fat are present in excess or when it accumulates due to poor health practices. During illness, weight may be lost due to the loss of water or protein and not due to a loss of unhealthy fat. In cases like this, weight loss may not necessarily be a good thing. It is important to distinguish between intentional weight loss and unintentional weight loss, such as that experienced by people who become ill. When the type of weight loss or reason for weight loss is not considered, people who lose weight may be more likely to experience poor health than those who do not lose weight.

Why is it that we believe that losing weight improves our health? Perhaps it is not the weight loss that causes changes in health for better or for worse, but the *processes* that cause weight loss that make the difference. When it comes to weight, we must be more specific in defining what we need or want to accomplish. Many or most of us need to gain the weight of muscle as much or more than we need to lose weight due to fat.

Perhaps weight loss shouldn't be thought of as a goal to be achieved in isolation. If we adopt healthier lifestyles, most of us will experience a loss of unnecessary fat and a building of healthy muscle. This will result in better body composition and less overall weight for most.

Genetics: If this is the "what" of weight, what is the "why" of weight? Why do I weigh what I weigh? Why do I have the body type or body composition that I have? We are taught that weight is simply the result of what we eat and what we burn up. (Calories in minus calories out determines your weight.) This is overly simplistic at best and inaccurate at worst. I prefer to look at weight as a reflection of one's makeup and one's environment.

There is no doubt that our genes play an important role in determining our health. There are debates about the relative role that genes and environment play in health and illness (nature versus nurture), but it is becoming more apparent that genes are not necessarily determinative. What we do may be as important as or more important than the genes that we inherit from our parents. This interplay of genetics and environment is often observed. Many of us know of families with one child who is obese and another who is not. You may have a coworker who seems to eat all of the time and not gain weight.

These examples speak to the genetic differences among individuals, as their inherited tendencies interplay with environmental factors. In order to get a better handle on health problems, particularly those related to weight, we must do a better job of addressing genetic uniqueness and variations among individuals. Since our genes determine how we respond to the environment, it makes sense that there will be differences among us when it comes to how we respond to exercise or different types of food. This is why it is impossible—or illogical—to recommend the same diet and exercise regimens to every individual and expect the same results. The results are as likely to be as varied as the differences in genetics and environment. The next time you see someone who has not been successful on a diet program, it may not be that they failed at the program—*the program may have failed them!* What happens to us can be determined by two factors: what we are born with and what we do with it.

Weight or, more appropriately, body composition should be seen not as a goal to be achieved but as a guide to use on the journey toward better health, a journey on which we are constantly trying to achieve and maintain a proper balance of muscle and fat and other factors important to our health.

What do you look like? Do you simply have too much fat, or do you need to increase your muscle mass? For many of us the answer is both. Yes, we know that we are overweight, but the main problem is that we are over-fat while at the same time being under-muscled. If this is the case, as we seek to improve our situation, our plan should not just center on weight loss. There are many ways to lose weight, but do these approaches address our main goals, which should be losing unnecessary fat, gaining muscle, and improving our health?

There are also those among us who are underweight and particularly lacking in muscle mass. This is very important in the elderly, in whom it has been shown that one of the major determinants of health is muscle mass, even among those who are not over-fat. So our major goal should not be to lose weight and be thin, but to improve our body composition and improve our overall health.

I would encourage you, therefore, to think of your weight as a guide that might give you some insight into your overall health rather than as a target to be achieved. A good weight or body mass index does not guarantee good health and fitness. After all, they make skinny caskets too!

Bottom line: Improving body composition matters more than losing (or gaining) weight.

Building Block #1: I will improve my body composition.

Action Step: Assess your body composition and devise a plan to improve it.

  Assess It:
   - Check height/weight table
   - Calculate body mass index
   - Calculate percent body fat using a scale, calipers or other measurement device
   - Calculate hip/waist ratio

  Use It Wisely:
   Once you have gotten a measure of your body composition, do not obsess over it. Remember, the measurements are just a guide that you can check periodically as just one measure of how you are doing. Do not consider them a necessary goal.

CHAPTER 2

NUTRIENTS

Carbohydrates

Stumbling Block #2: "Carbohydrates are bad for me."

As defined earlier, carbohydrates are the sugars, starches, and fiber that we consume. It is important to note that all carbohydrates are not created equal, and individual responses to carbohydrates are not the same.

If you have a metabolism or physiology that is predominantly geared toward carbohydrate conservation, a diet that is rich in carbohydrates and lacking in exercise can lead to increased fat production and subsequent obesity. But why does this happen?

James Neel, a geneticist, proposed the "Thrifty Gene Hypothesis" in 1962. The hypothesis is that many of us have genes that are adapted to a time and place in which carbohydrates were not present in abundance. For these people, the ability to quickly convert carbohydrates into fat for long-term storage would be an advantage. Theoretically, these individuals produce insulin readily in response to carbohydrate stimulation. This would certainly have been an advantage in a place and time in which carbohydrates were scarce, and when they were consumed, it was in the form of grains and other complex carbohydrates. This was especially true for females, who would need to be prepared to carry a pregnancy for almost a year and provide nourishment to the child through breast feeding for at least a year or two after that. The ability to convert carbohydrates readily to fat for storage in order to carry out these high-energy functions could help ensure survival of the group for another generation.

The presence of these genes in an environment of caloric and carbohydrate excess yields less optimal results. In these individuals, simple carbohydrates cause a rapid rise of insulin, sometimes to excess levels. In some, this insulin excess might cause a drop in blood glucose, possibly to subnormal levels. This "reactive hypoglycemia" drives an individual to consume carbohydrates in order to counteract the effects of the hypoglycemia, thus setting up a vicious cycle of gradually increasing insulin levels and increasing carbohydrate consumption. The result is ever-increasing energy storage as fat and eventual "down regulation" of receptor cells to the stimulus of insulin, so-called "insulin resistance." In this situation, genetically prone individuals are at risk for developing diabetes.

Correcting this scenario starts by realizing that some people are genetically programmed to produce insulin very efficiently in the presence of carbohydrate stimulation. Removal of the carbohydrate stimulus, especially simple or refined carbohydrates, is the mainstay of reversing this process. Decreased carbohydrate stimulation should lead to decreased insulin levels. Over time, the decreased insulin stimulation should allow peripheral receptor cells to reset and "up regulate" to the effects of insulin. How much reversal of this insulin resistance that can be accomplished may depend on an individual's genetics and how long and severely the process has been going on.

Exercise also plays a major role, especially activities that allow the muscles to empty themselves of glycogen (stored glucose), which then can be replaced from storage sources in the liver and dietary sources, decreasing the amount of carbohydrate that is stored as fat.

The dietary goal for dealing with this issue is to decrease consumption of simple, refined carbohydrates, which get into the bloodstream very quickly, while maintaining adequate levels of complex carbohydrates, which get into the blood stream slowly.

What does your diet look like? Is your diet overloaded by simple carbohydrates? Do you consume enough complex carbohydrates? The results of an imbalance in this area will vary from person to person. Some will experience an excess of weight, particularly abdominal weight. Some will experience an increased risk of developing other health problems, such as diabetes or problems related to having too little fiber in the diet. Some may not have many noticeable effects at all. However, the goal should be to improve this aspect of our diet as much as possible. For average Americans, I would expect that to mean increasing complex carbohydrates and decreasing simple, refined carbohydrates. How about you?

How much of a problem could this be for you? Diabetes, a family history of diabetes, abdominal obesity, multiple skin tags, diabetes during pregnancy, giving birth to large babies, and other symptoms can indicate genetic factors that can make it difficult to manage the consumption of large amounts of refined carbohydrates.

Bottom line: The type of carbohydrates that you consume is most important. Most of us consume too many simple carbohydrates and too few complex carbohydrates.

Building Block #2: I will consume the amount and type of carbohydrates best for me to improve my health.

Action Step: Assess your current carbohydrate intake and devise a plan to improve it.
Think about it—How much of your diet consists of refined carbohydrates, such as sugar, white bread, white rice cakes, cookies, candy, and soft drinks?
Improve it—Use a good-better-best approach. Artificial sweeteners and "diet" products may be better for you as a first step than using regular sugar and sugary foods and drinks. Natural sweeteners such as xylitol, stevia, agave, or natural honey may be a better next step as a transition from artificial sweeteners. Learning to appreciate natural flavors and using no sweeteners at all may be best for some foods and drinks.
Think about it—How much of your diet consists of complex carbohydrates, such as vegetables, fruits, and nuts?
Improve it—Again, use a good-better-best approach. Canned fruits and vegetables may be better than none at all. Frozen vegetables and fruits can be considered better than canned. Fresh vegetables and fruits are better than frozen. Local, organically grown fresh

fruits and vegetables may be best of all. Start with what is easiest for you and make improvements as you are able. Be sure to include in your diet additional sources of fiber such as cereals and beans.

Fats and Cholesterol

Stumbling Block #3: "Fat is bad for me."

Fats have been the dietary scourge of the past generation. Low-fat foods and diets abound. George Foreman has convinced us that draining the fat out of our meat as we cook it is a great thing to do. But is the bad reputation of fat a deserved one?

Let's begin by talking about the types of fats that are found in our diet. Fats have been divided into the basic categories of omega-3 (the so-called "good" fat) and omega-6 (the so-called "bad" fats). You will also hear talk of "trans fats." To understand the differences among these fats requires a discussion of just a bit of biochemistry.

Fats—or "fatty acids," as the scientists refer to them—actually perform several very important jobs in the body. In addition to being one of the major building blocks of the walls of all of our cells, fats are also an important source of energy for the body and serve as precursors to important chemicals.

Although we can make some fats, some we cannot make, and we must get them in the diet. The scientists call these "essential fats" or "essential fatty acids." These come in two basic chemical varieties: omega-3 and omega-6 (you may also see reference to products containing omega-9 fats, another variation on this theme). These names refer to the chemical links within the fat molecules that allow them to perform their unique functions.

You will also see fats referred to as "saturated" or "unsaturated." This is a chemical designation that refers to the number of hydrogen atoms on the fat molecule. One that is completely filled up with hydrogen is said to be saturated, and one that has one or more hydrogen atoms missing is said to be unsaturated.

In practical terms, saturated fats tend to be solid at room temperature, and unsaturated fats tend to be liquid. Saturated fats are considered by some to be bad because they have been associated with cardiovascular disease. This may not be absolutely true, however. Plant sources of saturated fat, such as coconut oil, are considered by some to be very healthful.

Fats are an important source of calories for energy production in the body. The omega-3 and omega-6 fats that we have discussed serve as important precursors for the chemicals that either cause or decrease inflammation in our bodies. In fact, a mismatch in the production of inflammatory versus anti-inflammatory chemicals may be important in the development of processes such as allergies, infections, and cancers. There is some discussion about what the proper ratio of omega-6 to omega-3 fats should be in our diet, but most authorities seem to settle around four to one. However, the American diet is said to have a ratio of about twenty to one omega-6 to omega-3. Dietary sources of omega-6 fats include processed meats, eggs, poultry, vegetable oils, and some nuts such as cashews. Omega-3 sources include some fish such as salmon, sardines and halibut, flax seeds, walnuts, and green vegetables such as broccoli, kale and spinach.

Everyone seems to agree that trans fats are bad. Trans fats are artificial fats that mimic natural fats. When the body tries to use these fats in the place of natural fats, damage can occur. This would be similar to trying to put a left-hand glove on your right hand.

Just as with fat, we have been led to believe that cholesterol is a bad thing. However, cholesterol is an essential, good thing. Cholesterol is an important component of cell walls and serves as the base upon which many hormones are built such as estrogen, testosterone, progesterone, and cortisol.

Even Low-Density Lipoprotein (LDL), the so-called "bad" cholesterol, is not completely bad. Only certain types of LDL cholesterol cause harm by collecting in the damaged linings of arteries. This damage is the real culprit when it comes to cardiovascular disease.

The body is capable of making most of the cholesterol that it needs. In fact, when you have your cholesterol measured, it has been estimated that approximately 80 percent of that measured level is due to what your body naturally makes and the rest is due to what you eat. A little-discussed phenomenon is that when you eat more cholesterol, your liver compensates by making less cholesterol. When you eat less, your body makes more.

Is an elevated cholesterol level a disease that needs to be cured, or rather a chemical marker for people who are more likely to develop cardiovascular disease? Why do we tell people that it is important to lower their cholesterol level? Lowering cholesterol has been shown to decrease the likelihood of developing cardiovascular disease. The question is whether *having* a low cholesterol is what causes the decreased risk, or whether the process of *getting* a low cholesterol measurement is important. It is possible to have a heart attack even with a normal cholesterol level.

High-Density Lipoprotein (HDL), the so-called "good cholesterol," has been associated with a decreased risk of developing cardiovascular disease. The job of HDL is to transport excess cholesterol from the body back to the liver. Although the native amount of HDL that we produce may be genetically determined, the level can be raised by exercise, supplements (i.e., niacin), and some medications.

The bottom line is that LDL and HDL cholesterol are both essential to our health. Statistically you can reap benefits from lowering your LDL cholesterol and raising your HDL cholesterol levels if they are out of the statistical range for your particular demographic. There are various calculators available that you can use to determine what your ideal cholesterol level should be. The goal then is to consume the correct proportion of fats, oils, and cholesterol to serve our needs.

Bottom line: Certain fats and oils are essential to a good diet, and not all saturated fat is bad. Cholesterol is important to the proper functioning of the body.

Building Block #3: I will consume the amount and type of fat that is best for me. I will also attain and/or maintain cholesterol levels that are appropriate for me.

> **Action Step:** Assess your current fat intake and devise a plan to improve it.
> **Think about it**—How much fat from pork, beef, shellfish, and poultry is there in your diet compared with fat from cold-water fish, such as salmon and mackerel, and vegetables?
> **Improve it**—Use a good-better-best approach. Start by trimming fat from beef, pork, and poultry before

consuming them. Better is to purchase lean cuts of meat rather than fatty cuts. Best is to consume limited amounts of grass-fed or organically raised meats, as well as seafood rich in omega-3 fats.

Proteins

Stumbling Block #4: "I eat meat so I get plenty of the best protein," or "I'm a vegetarian so I may not be getting enough protein."

We do not often think about differences among types and sources of protein. After all, when they are broken down into their constituent amino acids, does it really matter where they came from?

One of the primary purposes proteins serve is to supply us with essential amino acids. Just as with essential fats, we are not able to manufacture some amino acids, so they must be consumed in the diet. These are: isoleucine, leucine, lysine, methionine, phenylalanine, threoniine, tryptophan, and valine. Infants and growing children also need argentine, cysteine, histidine, and tyrosine. Don't worry about these names. The important thing is that we get the proper amount and type of dietary protein to assure we are getting the essential amino acids. Sources of protein in the typical American diet include dairy products (eggs, milk, cheese, yogurt), lean meats (fish, chicken, beef, pork) and plant sources such as beans, nuts (cashews, almonds, peanuts, pumpkin seeds, sunflower seeds), and grains (rice, wheat, corn).

Although proteins are not the major source of calories for most people, they can be used as a limited source of energy. More importantly, they serve as a source of structural components for the cells of the body. They also make up other essential components of the body, such as enzymes.

In this country, most of us get the majority of our protein from animal sources. However, plants can be a good source of protein, and those who eschew meats can still get plenty of good-quality protein from plant sources.

This is not to say that high-protein diets are favorable. Drastically increasing the total amount of protein that is consumed can cause problems (such as with the kidneys), particularly if enough water is not consumed. Proteins, particularly those from plant sources, are an important part of a well-balanced diet.

The goal then is to consume good-quality proteins and to be able to properly digest and absorb the proteins and amino acids in these foods.

Bottom line: Although meats are a main source of dietary protein, many of us in the United States would benefit from increasing plant sources of protein in our diet.

Building Block # 4: I will consume the amount and type of protein that is best for me from good-quality sources.

Action Step: Assess your current protein intake and devise a plan to improve it.

Think about it—How much protein in your diet is from animal sources such as beef, pork, and poultry compared with plant sources such as beans, peas, broccoli, spinach and brown rice?

Improve it—Use a gradual approach by incorporating more plant-based proteins into your diet while decreasing the quantity of animal-based proteins.

Vitamins and Minerals

Stumbling Block #5: "I need to take vitamin and mineral supplements in order to be healthy."

Who hasn't taken a vitamin at some time or another? Usually we do so because we think that it is a good idea to improve or maintain our health, or we try to use vitamins to remedy certain health issues. Sometimes vitamins are recommended to correct specific medical problems, such as anemia due to iron, $B_{12,}$ or folic acid deficiency.

A complete discussion of the vitamins and minerals that should be consumed by the average person is beyond the scope of this book; however, a brief discussion is in order. The best sources of vitamins and minerals are the foods that we consume, and theoretically we should be able to get all of the vitamins and minerals from our diet without the need for supplements. However, given the quantity of processed foods in our average diets and the farming practices that have stripped some land of needed minerals, even a good diet is not a guarantee of getting all of the vitamins and minerals that we need. For example, deficiencies of calcium and vitamin D are relatively common in the United States.

In as much as our commonly available foods are lacking in the vitamins and minerals that we need, supplementing is second best. There are many vitamin and mineral supplements that are available at just about any drug or grocery store in this country, but proper vitamin and mineral intake involves more than popping a bunch of pills. There is no easy way to completely determine exactly how much of every vitamin and mineral is needed by a given individual. Taking a multivitamin is a good way to cover the waterfront, but you must bear in mind that with this approach, you will be probably be getting more than is needed of some things, not enough of others, and just the right amount of some. In addition, the amount of any one vitamin or mineral that might be needed may change based on age, sex, medical condition, etc. Medical practitioners can employ a variety of tests to get an idea of particular nutrient deficiencies or excesses, but many may be missed. That being said, the day is rapidly approaching when we will be able to more completely determine the ideal amount of a comprehensive list of vitamins and minerals that might be needed by an individual at any given time.

The goal is to properly assess our individual vitamin and mineral needs and make sure that they are met through diet, supplementation, or a combination of the two.

Bottom line: Eating a proper diet and taking supplements may not guarantee sufficient consumption of the proper types and amounts vitamins and minerals.

Building Block #5: I will make an effort to determine and consume the proper amount and types of vitamins and minerals that I need.

> **Action Step:** Assess your current vitamin and mineral intake and devise a plan to improve it.
> **Think about it**—What natural sources of vitamins and minerals are there in your daily diet, including

those found naturally in fruits and vegetables as well as those found in fortified foods?

Improve it—Read labels and become familiar with the vitamins and minerals in the foods that you already consume. Consider adding a vitamin or mineral supplement, particularly if you have a specific need such as folic acid in pregnancy or calcium and vitamin D for those with osteoporosis (thinning bones).

Water

Stumbling Block #6: "I drink plenty of water."

"Water, water, everywhere, nor any drop to drink!" Or so it would seem if you look at the pessimists' view of water today.

Water could be considered the most vital factor for life as we know it. We all know that we need water, but how much? The traditional saying is that we all need eight eight-ounce glasses of water a day. As you probably realize by now, I don't believe in trying to put everyone into a one-size-fits-all box when it comes to health.

Sixty-four ounces might be a good place to start, but you may need more or less than that. If you are playing or working outdoors in the heat of the summer, you will obviously need more water than on a day that you spend indoors.

Our kidneys usually do a good job of getting rid of extra water. Most of us need only to be concerned with getting enough water. (I have, however, seen people who have become acutely ill from drinking too much water, so don't get too much of a good thing!) Some signs that you may not be getting enough water include feeling dry, weak, dizzy, or tired. More profound dehydration usually accompanies illness or heat exposure. Signs include mental status changes, fever, and seizures.

Short of this extreme, some people are chronically a quart low. Symptoms of mitral valve prolapse (such as palpitations) might be worse when blood volume is low. A concentrated-appearing urine and/or decrease in frequency of urination may accompany even mild dehydration. Hunger may also be a sign of needing water, not just food.

Although we can get much water from foods, particularly fruits and vegetables, we get most of our water from drinking. So, water is water, right? What is the big deal? For most of us, the source of water may not be as important as the quantity of water that we consume. However, if you are getting plenty of water in your diet, it may be time to consider the quality of water that you consume.

It is rare that we consume "pure" water. It almost always contains other chemicals or minerals, either by accident or design. Rain picks up chemicals from the atmosphere as it falls. Water from other natural sources (mountain runoff, lakes, rivers, streams, reservoirs, etc.) obviously gets mixed with other substances, both natural and man-made.

Tap Water. Our tap water, although drinkable, is not "pure." A list of impurities in your local tap water can be obtained from your water supplier. Although contaminants are kept within certain limits to render them harmless, you might want to go the extra mile to avoid overloading yourself with some of them. For example, some local water supplies contain detectable levels of minerals such as lead and copper, microorganisms such as bacteria and viruses, by-products of chemicals used to disinfect and decontaminate the water, and other chemicals that are added during water treatment or that find their way into the water supply in runoff from farms and factories.

Health departments throughout the country have divisions that are tasked with making sure that contaminants are kept to a minimum, and for most people in most locations, drinking tap water is fine and engenders no significant health detriments.

Bottled Water. Because of concerns about tap water, many drink bottled water. Although convenient, bottled water may not be any better than your local tap water. In fact, some bottled water is just processed tap water. Check with your local water department about the quality of your water to see if it is really any worse than bottled water.

Water Filtration. There are many water filtration systems available, from pitchers to whole-house systems. The filtration methods vary but usually involve a filtering agent such as charcoal. There are more sophisticated methods, such as reverse osmosis systems, but the goal is the same: to remove as many harmful things from the water as possible. If you know or think that your local tap water may contain some level of contaminants, a good water filter can help to improve the quality of your tap water even more.

The next issue is water quantity. The often-cited "eight eight-ounce glasses of water a day" may be an adequate starting place, but your specific requirements might vary significantly from this generality.

Medical conditions may also increase your need for hydration. Illnesses that cause vomiting or diarrhea will obviously increase your need to replace lost fluid. Fever also can cause a significant loss of water. Medications such as diuretics can cause loss of water from your system. Excessive caffeine or alcohol intake can also increase your need for water by causing you to expel more water.

Keep in mind that thirst is always a sign that you need water. Hunger may also mean that you need fluid. Dark, concentrated-appearing urine may indicate that your body is trying to hold onto water. Don't forget that a good supply of our daily water needs can be met through the foods, particularly fruits and vegetables. The goal is to consume an adequate amount of good-quality water on a daily basis.

Bottom Line: All water is not the same, but the differences may not be significant. The need for water can vary at different times among individuals.

Building Block #6: I will make sure that I get an adequate amount of water for me from the best sources, including food sources.

Action Step: Assess your current water intake and devise a plan to improve it.

Think about it—Do you find yourself stopping every time that you pass a water fountain, or do you frequently feel that you have a dry mouth or dry skin? Does your urine appear to be very concentrated or do you find yourself going for a long time without feeling the need to urinate?

Improve it—The average recommended water consumption is six to eight cups a day, but you may need more or less than this depending on your particular needs. You may need more working outdoors in the summer than when your days are spent indoors in the winter. Don't go overboard, but the kidneys generally do a good job of adjusting to the amount of water that you drink, so be liberal in your water consumption. Don't forget food-based sources of water, such as fruits and soups.

Calories

Stumbling Block #7: "I consume too many calories," or "Calories in minus calories out determines my weight."

Calories in minus calories out determines your weight, right? As you may have noticed from the foregoing discussion, the quality of calories rather than the quantity of calories may be more important for most of us most of the time. However, we do need to consume a certain amount of calories for proper functioning. The quantity of calories, however, may vary as much as the type of calories that we need.

There are several well-known stated amounts or formulas for determining desired caloric intake, but consider what may cause this number to vary for you. If the same amount of gasoline was put into a small car and a large truck, would they travel the same distance? Not likely. Gas mileage is determined by many factors, including the type of vehicle and the conditions under which it is driven.

The same can be said of us as individuals. Our caloric needs vary from time to time and from day to day. Likewise, what happens to those calories varies. There is not 100 percent absorption of the calories that are consumed, and what happens to those calories that are absorbed is not the same from person to person. This is why calorie counting, although useful, may not be an accurate or adequate way to determine or manage your specific calorie intake.

I often hear, "My problem is that I have too much of an appetite. I'm hungry all of the time. If I could control my appetite, I could lose weight." Although true, these statements may not be accurate. Hunger as a feeling or sensation may not be a signal that our bodies need or desire calories. It could be that our bodies need water or a specific nutrient. Hunger or craving may also indicate a desire for something other than food. Our language is replete with references such as, "food for thought," "thirst for knowledge," "I hunger for your love," etc.

Also, think about the language that we use when referring to our need for food. When we say, "I'm starving," or "I could eat a horse," we set ourselves up subconsciously to fulfill that need by eating a lot.

The next time you find yourself feeling hungry, think about the last time that you ate and consider whether you really need a lot of food. Perhaps you are hungry because it is time to eat, or you are bored and "hungry for adventure" or have a desire to fulfill a need that has nothing to do with food.

The goal is to consume an adequate number of good-quality calories to provide energy for our daily needs.

Bottom Line: It is important to get the proper quality as well as quantity of calories in the diet. Hunger may indicate a need for something other than calories (such as a nutrient, water, or a psychosocial need).

Building Block #7: I will consume enough of the best quality calories for me. When I am hungry, I will ask, "What am I hungry for?"

Action Step: Assess your current calorie intake and devise a plan to improve it.

Measure it—Most prepared, packaged, or processed foods now come with calorie information. You can use 2,000 calories a day as a benchmark, but keep in mind that your caloric needs may be more or less than this. If your daily activity includes a lot of physical activity, you may need more calories. Likewise, if your daily activity does not include as much physical activity (that is, you spend most of your day sitting), you may need fewer calories.

Improve it—If you are consuming more or fewer calories than you need, you can change it by changing the quantity of food that you consume, the quality of food that you consume, or a combination of each. The fat in food contains the most calories (9 calories per gram) while carbohydrates and protein contain less (4 calories per gram). Keep in mind, however, that your body metabolizes all of these nutrients differently, so the number of calories from one food may affect you differently than the same number of calories from another food. Think of 200 calories of ice cream compared with 200 calories of carrots.

CHAPTER 3

ACTIVITY

What we do is more important than what we are.

Physical Activities

Stumbling Block #8: "I must exercise in order to be healthy."

I am fond of telling my patients that exercise is not necessary in order to be healthy. Of course, this flies in the face of everything that they have been taught to believe, so they either give me a blank, disbelieving stare or ask me how this could be true. I tell the following true story.

Isabel, the Pedometer, and the Treadmill
We often make recommendations to patients regarding things to do in order to improve their health. I'm hesitant to ask anyone to do something that I wouldn't do myself, so I'm willing to try my own advice.

One recommendation is to use a pedometer to log the number of steps taken every day, with a goal of achieving at least 10,000 steps a day. *No problem*, I thought. *I'm on my feet all day working in an urgent care center. I'm sure that I get that many steps by lunch time. I'll get a pedometer, wear it all day, and show patients how easy it is to get ten thousand steps a day.* So, on went the pedometer. The first day I took 2,500 steps. I obviously did something wrong, so I moved the pedometer to the other hip. The next day, 2,300 steps. There had to be something wrong with the pedometer, but before I could get rid of it, my wife said that she would try it. She got 11,000 steps the first day.

"Eleven thousand! What did you do?!" I asked.

She casually responded, "I just went to the grocery store and did some shopping. You know, an average day."

I had to admit it wasn't the pedometer. It was me. I had woefully underestimated the amount of activity that I was getting every day. Not to be defeated, I decided to change the rules of the game. Instead of trying to get 10,000 steps a day, I would aim for a more modest 5,000 thousand steps. If I got 2,500 steps at work, I would get on the treadmill when I got home and get another 2,500 to equal 5,000. I would eventually increase the goal number of steps until I got to the magical 10,000 steps a day.

I was able to maintain this regimen with varying degrees of success for several weeks. Then hurricane Isabel hit the southeastern coast of the United States. As with the pedometer, I grossly underestimated what the hurricane would do to our area of Virginia. We had a large number of branches and leaves fall from the trees, making a shambles of what was left of our yard.

We also had no electricity for almost a week, which meant that I couldn't use my treadmill. It didn't matter, because I was in clean-up mode. I wasn't thinking about exercising. Out of habit, I continued to wear my pedometer. The first day of clean up, I got over 6,000 steps, and the second day over 8,000. *Well,* I thought, *if my goal was 5,000 steps and I got 6,000 steps, I don't need to exercise today.* In other words, exercise was *optional* that day because I had gotten my required number of steps by working in the yard rather than walking on the treadmill. I realized that separate exercise, which required putting on my tennis shoes and doing something extra, could be optional *every* day, as long as I could be active in other ways. In other words, it is not *exercise* that is important to health, but *activity. It is not exercise that most of us are missing in our daily lives, but activity.* If we would maintain an adequate level of daily activity, we would never need to set aside a special time to exercise. It would always be optional.

If we change our thinking from thinking about *exercise* to thinking about *activity*, a whole world of possibilities opens up. If you get out of the bed in the morning, you are active. In fact, sitting up in the morning and lying down at night constitutes one sit-up. And it counts! What if you did three or four of these sit-ups every day? That would be three to four times more activity than you are currently doing—and it counts!

Don't judge what you have to do or what is useful for you to do by some external or arbitrary standard that someone else has determined. Look at where you are now and see what you can do to improve. It doesn't have to be much to be significant, just a little more than you are doing now, then a little more, and a little more. A professional golfer probably wakes up every morning and asks, "What can I do today to become a better golfer?" The pro golfer may only make a small change in grip or stance, but that small change will be very significant to his or her overall success. We all have the same challenge. No matter how bad (or good) we are or have been, we can always do better. Moreover, we never finish. Success is not determined by completing certain tasks or reaching certain goals but by continuing to improve. "What can I do today to be a little more active?"

There are two basic types of physical activity (or exercise, if you feel more comfortable with that term). Aerobic activities are those that involve sustained or continuous movement, like walking, running, or swimming. These activities are called "aerobic" because the muscles predominantly work in such a way that they require oxygen. Anaerobic activities are resistance-type activities, such as weight lifting. They are called "anaerobic" because the muscles work in short bursts of activity that use energy without the use of oxygen.

So how do you know what to do? Think in terms of stamina (aerobic) and strength (anaerobic), and ask what you can do to improve each. What you will come to realize is that, although activities may be predominantly aerobic or anaerobic, enough of either will improve the other. For example, enough weight lifting will increase one's stamina, and enough walking will increase one' strength.

Do you have to join a gym or engage in a formal exercise program in order to succeed? Absolutely not! The only requirement is to look at the activity that you do now and devise a way to increase it. Remember the "in-bed sit-ups"? Another easy activity is to do twenty-five push-ups every day. "What?" you're asking. "I can't even do one push-up, and this guy is talking about doing twenty-five?! Can he possibly mean it?" Sure, I mean it. Don't lay prone on the floor on your knuckles and attempt to do twenty-five military-style push-ups. I'm not that crazy! Try facing a wall and standing a step or two away from it. Now reach forward, lean against the wall, and simply push away. Easy, right? Perhaps too easy. If so, step a little further from the wall and find a distance at which you can just do twenty-five (or whatever number that you choose) and keep doing your push-ups (or "push-aways") every day at that distance until it becomes easy. Then step out a little further, then a little further. You might have to move to using the back of a chair, a sink, etc. Eventually you will be doing push-ups on the floor with little more effort than it took to do the first twenty-five against the wall. It doesn't matter how long you have to do this before getting to the floor, or if you get there at all. The value of this activity is not in getting to a certain level of difficulty, but in doing a little more than you did before. And it all counts!

Mental Activities

Although we usually think of physical activity when it comes to exercise, the mind must also be exercised in order to attain and maintain optimal health. "Use it or lose it" applies to the brain as well as the body.

You probably know that the brain comes in two hemispheres, or halves. The left side predominantly controls logical, objective, and analytic thinking while the right side is responsible for creative, intuitive, and subjective thinking. If you are a mathematician or accountant, you are used to analytic thinking, whereas if you are a writer or artist, you do more creative thinking. Of course, these are extremes, and most occupations involve a combination of both types of thinking.

Regardless of what you are used to, it is helpful to exercise both sides of the brain. Crossword puzzles, chess, music, art, poetry, sports, and reading are examples of activities that can exercise the brain.

Social Activities

We all live in contact with others in communities of varying sizes. When performing social activities, we are usually in a position to be giving or receiving. It is important to do both in order to maintain a healthy social life.

Most of us have jobs that require us to be of service to others. Since childhood, we are taught the importance of helping others; however, it is equally important to be a gracious recipient of the service of others. Although we usually enjoy doing things for others, it is also important to feel appreciated.

It's also important to do things for ourselves. There are things that no one can do for us, and ignoring this aspect of our lives can lead to problems in other areas.

Building Block #8: I will continue to improve the amount and type of physical, mental, and social activities that I engage in to promote my health and wellness.

Action Step: Assess your current mental, physical, and social activities and devise a plan to improve them.
Think about it—What we *do* may be more important than what we *are*. Our daily activities are what shape us and change us from who we are into who we will be. "Change is inevitable, but growth is optional," as the saying goes. Are your activities working for or against you?
Improve it—Think of ways that you can improve your daily physical activity, particularly if your daily routine involves activities that require sitting for a long time. If you spend much of your time in physical activities, be sure to spend time pursuing activities that improve your mental health. Develop an appropriate balance of time spent with your friends and family.

Sleep

Stumbling Block #9: "I don't get enough sleep."

Sleep is recognized as an important determinant of health. Although we usually think of sleep in terms of how much that we get, we now know that the quality of sleep that we get is as important as, and in some cases more important than, the number of hours that we spend in bed. Lack of adequate sleep can lead to problems such as headaches and elevated blood pressure.

For many of us, getting a good night's sleep is not as easy as saying good night and closing our eyes. Restless leg syndrome and obstructive sleep apnea are examples of problems that can result in poor sleep. If you have a hard time falling asleep or staying asleep, or if you don't feel rested when you wake up, you may have one or more of these problems.

Some simple things that you can try in order to get a better night's sleep include going to bed at the same time every night and getting up at the same time every day (including weekends) or sleeping in a dark, quiet room and avoiding things that might stimulate you before going to bed such as exercise, caffeine, and alcohol. Some people find supplements such as melatonin or even a warm glass of milk to be helpful.

If you have tried these simple measures and still have more than occasional problems with your sleep, consider talking to your doctor about getting a formal sleep evaluation. These tests, usually performed in a sleep lab, can show problems such as sleep apnea or restless leg syndrome that interfere with sleep and can be treated.

Bottom line: Don't underestimate the role of getting proper sleep with regard to your overall health and wellness.

Building Block #9: I will try to improve the quantity and quality of sleep that I get.

Action Step: Assess your current sleep and devise a plan to improve it.

Think about it—Are you getting a good night's sleep? Do you feel tired when you wake up in the morning? Do you feel the need to take naps? Do you snore loudly or has anyone told you that you stop breathing when you sleep?

Improve it—If you answer yes to these questions, you could have a significant sleep disorder. Talk with your physician about this. If you occasionally have problems with sleep, follow the tips for improving your sleep hygiene. You might also consider temporary use of over-the-counter medications or herbal supplements.

CHAPTER 4

STRESS

What's eating you is as important as what you are eating.

Stumbling Block #10: "I'm too stressed out!"

One way to think of the nervous system is in terms of its voluntary and involuntary parts. The voluntary nervous system is the part that we can consciously control. The involuntary part functions automatically, without us having to make a conscious effort to control it. There is some overlap between these two systems. Our breathing is mostly involuntary, but we can consciously control it, at least to a certain extent.

When it comes to our health, we usually think about the things that we do voluntarily, such as engaging in physical activities. We don't often think about the role that the involuntary or autonomic nervous system (ANS) plays in our overall health. The ANS controls heart rate and blood pressure, breathing, and intestinal functions, for instance. Because these activities take place automatically, we aren't often aware that they are taking place—until something goes wrong. Then we might experience an involuntary cough or nausea and vomiting. The voluntary nervous system even becomes involved when we experience chills and shivering.

There are two main parts of the ANS: the sympathetic nervous system and parasympathetic nervous system. There are exceptions, but in general, the sympathetic nervous system speeds up functions such as breathing, heart rate, and blood pressure, and the parasympathetic system slows things down and is involved in digestion. The adage is that the sympathetic system is involved in "fight or flight" responses, and the parasympathetic system is involved when we need to "rest and digest."

The "fight or flight" response gets its name from the fact that its purpose is to prepare our bodies for times of physical emergency, such as being threatened by a vicious animal. In those circumstances, we need to be able to fight off the attacker or run away to safety. This requires an increase in muscular activity and mental alertness. Our system has to rev up. In addition to the nervous system response, our body releases stress hormones such as adrenaline and cortisol into the blood stream. These hormones further increase nervous system activity and release sugar into blood stream for energy. Although these responses cause great changes in the system, they can be lifesaving in an emergency.

In the caveman days, threats were usually physical, short lived, and intermittent. The problem in our modern society is that we are faced with threats that are mental, long lasting, and chronic. We may think of the threats or stressors in our lives as just being the big obvious ones, but we are also faced with smaller, less noticeable threats that nonetheless have a significant impact on our well-being. We wake up to the alarm clock, fight traffic on the way to work, deal with all of the individual stresses at work, etc. Each of the small stressors induces a small stress response, from which we rarely have time to recover before the next one occurs. Our sympathetic nervous systems are often overcharged and overworked.

The parasympathetic nervous system is involved with digestion and slowing of some functions, such as heart rate and blood pressure. Under normal circumstances, this part of the nervous system balances the sympathetic system and allows functions such as digestion to occur while allowing the rest of the body to rest.

One way to actively stimulate the parasympathetic nervous system and dampen the sympathetic nervous system is through controlled breathing. Whether it's sports, martial arts, yoga, or meditation, all use breathing to shift the nervous system into a more parasympathetic state and put the body and mind into a more calm and relaxed state. When it's time to take a break, we talk of "taking a breather." In fact, relaxed breathing may be a major factor in the satisfaction that people get from smoking.

If you would like to try it for yourself, one simple method is to very slowly breathe in, hold it, breathe out, and hold it. Do this active relaxation for short periods during the day, even if only for a minute, to counteract the small recurrent stress responses that you experience during the day.

Many excellent sources are available to teach you more specific, useful methods for using breathing and relaxation techniques. I would encourage you to investigate these and make this a routine part of your health and wellness efforts.

Building Block #10: I will reduce the effects of stressors in my life by actively relaxing and engaging in other stress relieving activities.

Action Step: Assess your current stress level and devise a plan to improve it.

Think about it—Everyone has stressors in their lives. How are you managing yours? Do you manage family and work obligations and problems without undue difficulty? Do you often feel overwhelmed?

Improve it—Ask for help and spread the load when you can, both at home and at work. Try not to be concerned that others will think less of you for doing so. Develop mental and physical outlets outside of the home and workplace that allow you to relax or blow off steam. Seek professional help from a counselor or psychologist if you find it hard to cope.

CHAPTER 5

Environmental Factors

Stumbling Block #11: "There is nothing that I can do about my environment."

We have been aware of the dangers of pollution of our air, water, and soil since the onset of the industrial revolution. Although few would dispute the presence of such factors, how much influence they might have on us is the source of seemingly endless debate.

Even though we may not be able to accurately quantify the effect of the multitude of pollutants that we might be exposed to over a lifetime, it does no harm to be aware of what is out there and to do our best to minimize our exposure and the effects of such exposure.

Air Quality

It might seem that we have little control over the quality of air to which we are exposed. After all, breathing is a necessity, regardless of the quality of air that is available. We may not be able to do much about the greater problem of air pollution on a worldwide basis, but we can work through our local legislators, communities, and industries to support legislation and other measures that help to improve the overall quality of air to which we are all exposed. We can also make the decision to minimize our own individual contributions to this problem by trying to drive cars that are less polluting, minimizing our use of aerosols, etc.

We may actually have more power to control the quality of air within our homes. Indoor air pollution is probably an underappreciated but significant source of pollutants that can be controlled and minimized.

This includes indoor pollutants such as: cigarette smoke, candles, gasses from new carpeting, etc. The amount of indoor pollutants obviously varies with location, and you might find more or less in your home. Measures such as using air filters and keeping houseplants can go a long way to reducing the amount of these indoor pollutants.

Food Quality

One reason that humans have been able to thrive in society is the ability of our societies to feed us. Modern farming techniques have allowed fewer farmers to feed more people. Soil treatments are used to replace nutrients stripped from the soil, and pesticides and herbicides are commonly used for our plant sources of foods. Animal sources of food have also been affected by aggressive practices that provide more animals to feed more people.

However, we are now seeing the downside of these agricultural practices. We know that the chemicals found in insecticides and pesticides accumulate in the food chain. These substances enter our bodies both directly when we use them and indirectly when we eat the plants and animals that were exposed to them.

The steps that take place to deliver our food to us include harvesting, transportation, processing, and storage. These also affect food quality. It is now easier to avoid some of these detriments by buying locally grown foods from farmer's markets, by consuming organic foods, or by growing your own fruits, vegetables, and herbs. Check to see what is available in your local community.

Caffeine, Sweeteners

You have probably heard the debates about alcohol, caffeine, and artificial sweeteners. Depending on what you read, you may believe them to be the worst things that you can consume or that they are relatively harmless substances.

Although it is true that these substances can cause problems, they are not equally bad for everyone. How bad they are for you may depend on your genetics and your lifetime exposure to these and other, similar substances. Caffeine is naturally found in many plants, but overconsumption from natural or artificial sources can cause problems ranging from jitteriness and insomnia. They can also affect the body's ability to metabolize other substances, such as medications. Some people are born with genetic differences that make it more difficult to handle chemicals found in some artificial sweeteners. For these people, avoiding artificial sweeteners can be important. This does not mean going without. Artificial sweeteners can be replaced with products containing xylitol or stevia.

If you have issues with your health or just want to maximize your wellness, see what happens when you decrease or eliminate these substances from your diet. You might be surprised!

Alcohol, Drugs, Toxicants

Anything that we ingest in order to cause a change in the body could be considered a drug. Traditionally, these drugs have been substances found in the environment, particularly plants, that were noted to have beneficial effects. In modern times, we have been able to develop drugs designed to cause specific changes or provide particular benefits when they are taken.

The body often considers these substances to be poisons or toxins, and after we ingest them, it sets out to try to rid itself of them. This detoxification takes place primarily in the liver. Pharmacologists can now design drugs that take these systems into account and sometimes develop a drug that doesn't become activated until it is processed by the body.

Although much research goes into the development of our currently available medicines to ensure their safety and efficacy, anything that we ingest can cause problems, either due to the nature of the drug itself or due to the particular person taking them or a combination of the two. Anything that we consume can not only cause the desired change but also side effects, changes that we don't want. In this regard, there should be no distinction between pharmaceuticals and so-called natural drugs or supplements. Too much of anything can be bad, and individuals can have adverse reactions to any given substance. Be wary when something is advertised as being "safe" or "natural" with "no side effects." It is unlikely that there is any substance that is so specific that it only does one thing when it is ingested. The only way that a substance can have no side effects is to have no effects.

Should drugs and supplements be avoided at all costs? Absolutely not. Consider them tools to be used to bring about a desired change in your body, to alleviate some discomfort, remedy some disease or dysfunction, or assist the body in doing what it needs to do.

There are also substances that are considered toxic in all instances, or "toxicants." Technically, anything can be toxic in too great a quantity; however, I am referring to things that we would not intentionally ingest because they serve no useful function in the body. This includes ingestion of substances that might contaminate foods, such as insecticides or pesticides, and exposure to harmful substances in the environment, such as lead or mercury.

Ever since man began consuming and fermenting plants, he has known about the mind-altering potential of these substances. It is well documented that moderate consumption of some types of alcohol, such as red wine, can confer health benefits. But there are also potential detriments that can come from overconsumption or addiction. The same can be said of prescription drugs, whether they be narcotics (e.g. pain medications such as codeine), amphetamines (such as Ritalin), or other medications. They do serve useful purposes when used appropriately, but there must always be recognition of the potential for overuse, misuse, or abuse.

Electromagnetic/Radiation Factors

A complete discussion of electromagnetic radiation is beyond the scope of this text, but it does deserve mention. Whether it's cell phones, microwave ovens, television, power lines, or x-ray machines, we are surrounded by man-made sources of radiation. This is in addition to the natural sources of radiation that we are exposed to, such as the sun.

Although it is known that radiation is detrimental, how much it takes to harm an individual and under what circumstances can be a source of controversy. For example, can exposure to the radiation from a cell phone cause problems? The answer might technically be yes, but is anyone exposed to a strong enough dose for a long enough period of time to cause problems? We may not be able to answer these questions at this time, but limiting our exposure to any of these sources of radiation is a wise precaution.

There are several products for sale that claim to be able to manipulate the body at the electromagnetic level or mitigate the harm from environmental electromagnetic radiation. There is little objective, reproducible evidence that documents the benefit of such devices, but there is also little evidence of harm.

Microorganisms and Parasites

Microorganisms like bacteria and viruses existed on this planet long before the first humans came to be. We are familiar with those that cause problems, such as the flu virus and the Salmonella bacterium, but there are many that are not harmful and some that are beneficial. Parasites include larger organisms that can live in us, such as worms and single-cell organisms, and those that live on us, such as scabies.

We now live in a time in which antibiotic, antiviral, antiparasitic, and antifungal medications can be used to help rid ourselves and our environment of harmful microorganisms. These can by their nature be harmful to our system, particularly when overused. We also have to keep in mind that we are also dependent on beneficial bacteria to coexist with us and help maintain our health. There is now a common knowledge of the need to decrease our use of antibiotics and to increase our exposure to beneficial bacteria, known as probiotics.

The goal is to strike a balance between what we actively do to manage the microorganisms and parasites in our environment and supporting the body in its natural ability to deal with these organisms when we encounter them.

Positive Environmental Influences

The foregoing factors can be considered negative influences, and we want to minimize our exposure to them. There are also positive factors that should be included, like vitamins and minerals, and environmental factors such as sunshine. Although these can be harmful in too great a quantity, we can also have problems if we do not get enough of them.

Building Block #11: I will reduce the effects of negative environmental factors and increase positive environmental factors in my life.

Action Step: Assess negative and positive environmental factors and devise a plan to improve them.

Think about it—No one lives in a perfect world, but do you face particular challenges in yours? Do you spend a significant amount of time in a car? Are you regularly exposed to radiation or chemicals in workplace? Do you live in an area of significant air, water, or soil pollution? Do you consume significant amounts of processed foods, and do your foods contain adequate amounts of vitamins and minerals?

Improve it—Do your best to decrease your exposure to chemicals in the air, water, and food. Consider using vitamin or mineral supplements if you have a deficiency. Consider using air and water filters in your home and workplace. Drink plenty of water. If you must use insecticides, pesticides, or other chemicals in your work or home, do your best to protect yourself by using gloves, protective clothing, and a respirator or mask. Wash your skin, hair, and clothing frequently to prevent prolonged or recurrent exposures.

PART II

BEYOND THE PHYSICAL

CHAPTER 6

THE FAMILY & COMMUNITY

Stumbling Block # 12: "My success is entirely up to me," or "My failure is entirely my own fault," or "My family and friends are holding me back."

"No man is an island," as the saying goes. Unless you are literally living on an island by yourself, you are part of a community. In fact, you are probably a member of several communities. How you relate to these communities and how they relate to you has much to do with your successes and failures in life.

We often discount the influence of our family on our personal health. We inherit the genes of our ancestors, but we also accumulate habits and cultural norms as we live our lives. For example, if your ancestors come from the American South or the Orient or the Caribbean, you are more likely to consider rice an integral part of your daily dining. The same goes for cooking styles (such as deep frying) and even the time of day that you eat. I remember being totally confused as a child visiting my grandmother in Louisiana and having to eat dinner at two in the afternoon! We were used to eating our largest meal much later in the day. We must keep in mind that many of our family traditions were developed in times when they were useful or even essential for survival.

We should think of our family, both immediate and extended, as a source of information, motivation, and inspiration. This may be easier in some families than others, but all of us have received something from our family, even if it's nothing more than genes. It is up to us to determine how we capitalize upon that inheritance. In order to do this, we must first realize that there is a problem. Next, the problem has to be specifically identified. Then a plan to correct the problem must be created, and finally that plan must be executed.

I recall an overweight patient who struggled to get her body composition under control. Over the period of a year, however, she made remarkable progress. What happened during that year? Her husband was diagnosed with diabetes! Suddenly *they* had to watch what *they* ate and *they* had to increase *their* activity level. Since he was now involved, she became successful.

According to our model, she realized that there was a problem because she was overweight. However, when she identified the role that her husband played in her daily activities and choices, she was able to create a different plan for success that now included him. Together, they were able to execute that plan, leading to success for both of them.

Stumbling blocks to success at this level include location, association, cooperation, commitment, and cost. You might create a plan that includes daily walking, but you might live in an area in which this is difficult due to geography, weather, safety, or other factors. You might plan to include your associates in your plan, but they may be reluctant to participate. Even if they do participate, their level of commitment may not be the same as yours, and their participation may soon fade away. There is a cost to making any change. The cost may be monetary—like the price of better quality food or a gym membership—the cost of time, or even the cost of a strain on relationships. Some of our associates may resent the fact that we want to change for the better, especially if those changes impact their world, such as making the choice to spend time at the gym rather than spending time with them in front of the television.

In order to overcome these obstacles we must be willing to communicate, negotiate, and collaborate. We can't assume that those in our social circles know or even care what we are trying to do when it comes to our health and wellness. The better a job that we do in communicating our needs and desires, the better the chance that they will be supportive of our endeavors. Even if they want to help, it may not be on our terms. We must be willing to negotiate—give and take—in order to enlist their help. We must also remember that it is not their help that we want in doing something for us, but their cooperation in doing something with us—that is, collaboration.

Remembering that we are a part of several communities gives us the opportunity to take advantage of many available resources—family, friends, and neighbors—who can play an integral part in our journey to optimal health and wellness.

Building Block #12: I will let my family and community be a part of my success.

Action Step: Assess your current family and community relationships and devise a plan to improve them.

Think about it—"No man is an island," as the saying goes. We live, work, and play with others. Are your relationships with others healthy and uplifting, or are they unhealthy and destructive? Do you tend to be a loner without close friends or family?

Improve it—Social outlets do not need to be numerous to be significant. A few good relationships can be better than many poor ones. Consider getting involved in organizations that allow you to support others and give back. Do not take your family members for granted. You may not have chosen them, but you can foster relationships with them that are good for you and them.

CHAPTER 7

THE INNER SELF

Stumbling Block #13: "Everything that I need for success is 'out there.'"

When considering failure at other levels, whether it is failure to attain or maintain optimal health or optimal relationships, the roots of these failures can almost invariably be found at (or reflected in) this basic fundamental level. Philosophers and theologians spend their lives trying to understand this aspect of the human condition; I won't pretend to be able to cover it all here, but there are some basic aspects that are important to consider when it comes to our health.

As with the other levels, we must first realize that problems exist, identify what those problems are, create a plan for improvement, and execute that plan. Factors that can alter the chance of success include: aspiration, inspiration, motivation, dedication, and cost.

At this level, we must first aspire to change. You may have seen someone in what you might consider to be deplorable circumstances, but they appear to be perfectly happy. This may be because they have no aspiration or desire for things to be different. But before you begin to feel sorry for someone else, keep in mind that someone else may look at your circumstance the same way.

Even if someone aspires to do better, they sometimes fail to take action. But they might be inspired to take action. We often look for inspiration in our lives. We have heroes and read stories of others who have overcome difficult circumstances. These are not enough. We must also be motivated to make a change. This may actually be the most important factor with which to contend. We may be mentally or spiritually be prepared to make a change, but we must also be inspired enough to actually take action.

After we begin to make a change, we must continue that change. There must be a dedication to the change that was made and a commitment to continue in the new direction.

And as always, there is a cost. It is not always easy to let go of our old selves and take on the role of the new self, but this is what is necessary in order to improve our health and wellness.

The Regis Question and the Person in the Mirror
A few years ago, Regis Philbin hosted a popular television show called *Who Wants to Be a Millionaire?* Contestants answered a series of questions of increasing difficulty in an attempt to win one million dollars. But what if winning a million dollars didn't involve asking questions? What if Regis said, "Here is a million dollars. All you have to do is _____ [fill in the blank: exercise daily, forgo gratuitous sweets, etc.] for a month." Could you do it? I would have to be honest and say, "Yes, I could do it. I could exercise every day for a month if it meant receiving one million dollars at the end of that time." But then I would have to look at the man in the mirror and say, "So why am I not doing it? Are my health and life not worth the same effort as receiving a million dollars?" Tough questions. The answers are critical to understanding what makes us click and ultimately determine our success or failure.

The Reverse Traffic Light (Go on Red)
Psychologists talk about the concept of "locus of control." Are we motivated by external factors or by internal factors? In fact, we are controlled by both, but one usually dominates more than the other in certain circumstances. If you are driving your car through an intersection, these factors are at work. There is the internal motivation of reaching your destination sometimes competing with the external factors that control traffic flow. If the light is green, there is no external reason to slow down or stop. You *could* slow down because you notice that the light has been green for some time and is likely to change. If the light is yellow, you *should* slow down, and you *could* come to a stop in anticipation of the light changing to red. When the light is red, you *must* stop.

This "could, should, must" paradigm often prioritizes our lives, particularly if we are more motivated by external factors. Have you ever paid your taxes on April 15? You *could* pay them by February 15, you *should* pay them by March 15, but you *must* pay them by April 15. Have you ever pulled an all-nighter to finish a term paper for school or a project for work? Most likely, you *could* have finished it two weeks earlier, you *should* have finished it a week ago, but you *must* finish it now.

"So I wait until the last minute. If it gets done by the deadline, what's the problem?" If this happens occasionally, well that makes you human like the rest of us. But if this is your routine, it may speak to underlying factors in your personality. Waiting until the last minute or until circumstances dictate that you *must* act is the ultimate way of putting the ball in your court. Who hasn't been by themselves on the basketball court and pretended to be making the last, winning shot in the championship game? I don't think that there is anything necessarily wrong with this, but how many times can you run through the yellow light before you end up running the red light and having an accident?

The underlying physiology in these circumstances is the stress response, a release of adrenaline and other stress hormones, stimulation of the sympathetic nervous system, and that feeling of excitement. This adrenaline rush is a fine thing when it results in what it was designed for, a burst of physical activity that results in resolution of the stressful situation, the fight or flight response.

For some, this excitement feeds into emotions that actually make them feel good. For others, it causes feelings of fear or dread. In other words, we are looking to feel good and/or avoid feeling bad. If you are one who likes this feeling, you might be driven to actually seek situations that will allow you to feel this, even if you are not consciously aware of it.

For many of us in today's world, our stressful situations are often more mental than physical. Even though we are motivated to take physical action, the action required is usually not running as fast as possible for as long as possible or literally fighting for our lives. Most of the time we are faced with small frequent stressors during the day: wake up to the alarm clock, listen to the morning news, fight traffic on the way to work, deal with all of the stressors at work. You get the idea. Each one of these events represents a mini fight or flight response. The response, although not as vigorous, is the same. Over the years, this chronic stimulation might eventually contribute to the development of hypertension and other cardiovascular diseases, diabetes, anxiety, depression, and other health problems.

By the way, why do you use an alarm clock? It's obviously to keep from oversleeping. But do you remember as a child needing an alarm clock to wake you up on Christmas morning or on your birthday? Even now, how often do you find that you wake up before the alarm clock on the day of vacation or some other significant event? These are times when you feel that you *must* get up.

So how do we change things to improve our health? It is beyond the scope of this book to discuss changing one's locus of control from external to internal (or vice versa), but the idea is to change those "coulds" to "shoulds" and those "shoulds" to "musts." This might be as simple as literally changing our language when we think about or discuss our actions. "I should work on my project now, even though it is early," rather than "I could work on my project now, even though it's early." Or better yet, "I must work on that project now because it is early!" How? Where there is a will, there is a way. Anything that we can do now to avoid a more stressful situation in the future and decrease the cumulative effects of stress in our lives is worth doing.

Why do we fail? There are plenty of books and programs that tell us what to do, when to do it, and how to do it. Some even tell us why we should change, so why are we still failing? Perhaps because we are a goal-oriented society. Our goal is to have a goal. Our plan is to have a plan. "To fail to plan is to plan to fail!" You have heard all of this before and have probably tried all of this before. But maybe the problem is that we always embark on these health improvement adventures with the goal of meeting some goal—a certain weight, a certain blood pressure, a certain blood sugar, a certain dress size, etc. "Ay, there's the rub." If having a concrete goal and a well thought-out plan were all that defined success, we would all be more successful than we have been. Every team has the same goal and each has an excellent game plan, but only one emerges as a winner.

Perhaps for ourselves, it is time that we changed our focus from goals to process. In other words, instead of having a goal of losing a certain amount of weight, we could make a decision to improve the process of living—eating a little better; improving our activity type and level; adjusting our social network to one that supports us better. We will never completely achieve any of this to perfection, and that's the point. Instead of trying to reach a certain place, we should be happy with our current place and work to improve ourselves little by little, day by day. Babies don't learn to walk with the goal of getting from one place to another. Their goal is to walk simply because they can, simply for the pleasure of doing it. We might likewise do better if we made it our commitment to do better just for the sake of doing better without any ulterior motive, but just because that's what we are meant to do.

Education

"Knowledge is power," but it is more than a matter of pure knowledge. If I know all of this, why doesn't my tie hang down quite as straight as it should? I believe it is because many of us have never taken the time to really learn about what makes us tick or how we work. The basic process for understanding how we work physically is education. We touch on much of this in this book, but there are many resources available for more in-depth study. The important thing is to do it and not assume that we know or understand everything that there is to know.

Studying what makes us work mentally, emotionally, socially, and spiritually is not something that we routinely do in the Western world. Reflection, meditation, and prayer are ways to educate ourselves about ourselves.

Reflection/Meditation/Prayer

There are some things about ourselves that are not to be found in books, both questions and answers. Why am I the way that I am? Why do I do the things that I do? At one level, these rhetorical questions will have no concrete answers and will continue to be discussed by philosophers. At another level, these are practical questions that can lead to practical answers. At this level, asking the right question or being able to ask the right question is as important, if not more important than, being concerned with coming up with the right answer.

Although there are useful external processes that we can use to aid in this process, the key is to find a way to search ourselves for the answers. Many cultures have formal methods of self-exploration, such as mediation or prayer. Although these are very good and very useful techniques, simply taking the time to sit back quietly and reflect on our strengths and weaknesses can also yield results.

Building Block #13: Everything that I need for success is "in here."

Action Step: Assess your current knowledge and motivations and devise a way to improve them.

Think about it—Solomon Short said, "Half of being smart is knowing what you're dumb about." This book is not intended to give you all of the answers but to prompt you to ask better questions. In what areas do you need more knowledge or experience? Do you have adequate motivation or reasons for wanting to make changes in your life?

Improve it—Use this book as a jumping-off point to research areas that are important for you to change at this time. There are many quality resources available at your local library, bookstore, and on the Internet. Consider talking to people whom you know that are successful in areas in your life that you would like to improve. These could include friends, family, coworkers, and professionals.

PART III

PUTTING IT ALL TOGETHER

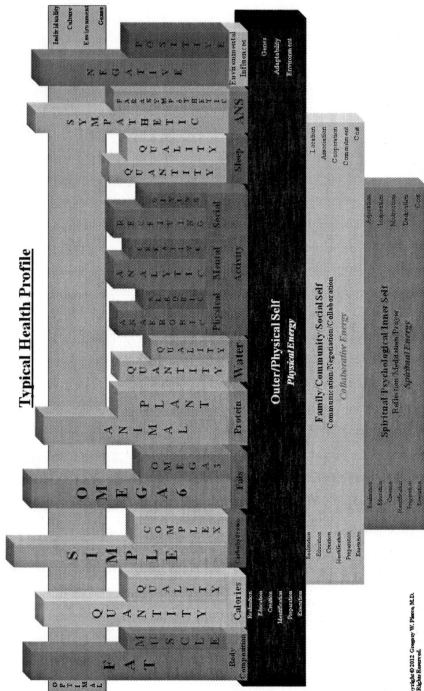

CHAPTER 8

THE PIERCE RECIPE

Does Knowledge Equal Success?

Knowledge of this information is good but not sufficient for our success. Realization is the first step. We must realize that we have problems, challenges, or a need or ability to do something better. Sometimes it is just the realization that we could be better off than we are now. After this realization comes the identification of the specific areas in which changes can and should be made. A plan for change must then be created and successfully executed.

These steps may seem easy and straightforward, but success can depend on several factors. First, our genetics determines a great deal of our potential and how our body will change or adjust when we try to make changes. Although genes may not determine the outcome in all cases, they can make changes easier or harder to accomplish. Genes also partially, but not completely, determine our adaptability, which is our ability to adjust to changes in our environment. This could be our internal physical environment, our external physical environment, or our social environment. Our environments are very important in determining if and how we change.

Knowledge does not necessarily equal success. Knowledge must be applied in specific ways, with a mind toward turning stumbling blocks into stepping stones on the way to success.

It is relatively easy to give a list of factors such as the ones discussed thus far and simply say, "Make it right!" But what does it mean to "make it right," and how do these factors relate to each other?

When looking at a factor such as body fat composition or carbohydrate consumption, the premise is that for any given individual, an optimal range exists. This optimal range is determined by several factors, including our genes (what we are born with), our culture and environment (what we learn based on where and with whom we happen to live), and our own individual likes and dislikes.

These factors have been organized into a profile called the **PIERCE RECIPE**. What does this mean? PIERCE refers to a Personal Inventory of Everything Relevant, Changeable, and Executable.

When looking at factors important to our health and life, they should be **Personal**. It is easy to find information written by, for, and about other people, but how does that information apply to you? This book should give you ways in which to consider each of these factors in a way that applies to you.

This is an **Inventory,** or accounting of the factors important to you at this time. This is not meant to be an all-inclusive list, and you should feel free to add or subtract items to fit your personal situation now and as it changes. Think of this inventory as a dynamic list that changes as you change.

Does this really mean **Everything**? Perhaps not in the literal sense, but every kind of thing should be included in this inventory, including what you eat, your activities, and your relationships with others, to name a few. Many currently available sources of information fall short because they fail to consider one or more of these areas that might be important for a given individual.

Likewise, the information or factor in the inventory should be **Relevant**. Sure, something may be true and may apply to other people, but is it a practical consideration for you and your situation right now?

It should also be **Changeable**. It may be a nice academic exercise to consider all sorts of scientific factors that affect our bodies and health, but if you can't change them at this time, the consideration becomes impractical. That's not to say that you won't be able to change a given factor in the future, even if it is not possible to do so now.

Finally, the changes must be **Executable**, or at least a good-faith effort should be possible. Something might be good to change in the long term, but if our current situation precludes the ability to make such a change, that factor should be postponed until it is practical to change it.

You can use the chart to look at your current situation and determine if you are above, below, or within that ideal range. Getting the factor into the optimal range turns the stumbling blocks into building blocks.

For example, looking at Body Composition (a term I prefer over "weight"), many of us are "under-muscled" and "over-fat." The goal is not to simply lose weight, but instead to increase muscle mass and decrease unnecessary fat.

If you are like many of us, your diet is overloaded with simple carbohydrates while being deficient in complex carbohydrates. Likewise, most Americans have a diet that consists of too many omega-6 fats compared to a relative lack of omega-3 fats.

Consumption of adequate protein is not a problem for most of us; however, we might enhance our health by increasing plant protein in our diet and decreasing (and improving the quality of) animal sources of protein.

Calorie consumption is not a problem for many of us, but if we use the foregoing strategies, we can improve the quality of calories that we consume while reducing the overall amount of excess calories. Likewise, improving the quality of water that we consume is as important as making sure that we consume an adequate amount of water.

I have already discussed using the term "activity" rather than "exercise" to describe what we need to do physically as well as mentally and socially. With our typical American lifestyle, most of us would benefit from increasing activity in most or all of these areas.

Sleep is something that we don't often consider when it comes to our health, but an adequate quantity and quality of sleep are essential to enhancing our health.

Stressors are a constant factor in life, but we can choose how we deal with them. We can engage in activities that increase our relaxation reactions and decrease our stress reactions.

There are a myriad environmental factors, both internal and external, that have positive and negative influences on our health. The goal is to identify those factors, then increase the positive ones and decrease the negative ones.

Being aware of these factors is necessary but not sufficient to successful health enhancement. We often fail to make adequate progress toward our goals because of our social situation, which includes the people and situations that support us or hinder us. Improvements in our family and community life help to support all of our efforts toward physical improvement.

Even with a clear understanding of what we need to do physically and having adequate social support, if we are not able to understand those internal factors that make us tick, we will not understand the most fundamental factors that are responsible for our success.

RECIPE refers to the components necessary to make a successful change: **R**ealization, **E**ducation, **C**reation, **I**dentification, **P**reparation, and **E**xecution.

We must **Realize** that a problem exists or that a change is needed. For example, we have to realize that our current diet may be causing problems before we can attempt to change it.

Once we realize that there is a problem, we must **Identify** exactly what the problem is and **Educate** ourselves to know exactly what the problem entails and what it will take to make an improvement.

The next step is the **Creation** of a plan to make the needed changes. This is often easier said than done. Modeling others can be helpful, but keep in mind that adaptations often have to be made in order to make someone else's plan work for you.

Preparation is often overlooked when it comes to making changes. For example, a goal might be to increase aerobic activity, but what does it mean? More running, more walking, a membership at the gym? When will I find time for these activities? Do I have the proper equipment? The devil is always in the details, and without proper preparation, the stage is set for failure.

When it comes to **Execution,** "the best laid plans of mice and men . . ." You know the saying. How often have we succeeded in the other steps but failed to execute properly? This can be the most difficult step for some of us, but also the most rewarding. If we are properly educated, motivated, and prepared, execution is much easier.

Even when all of these things are done optimally, there will still be differences in results among individuals. What accounts for the differences? At the physical level, it starts with our genetic uniqueness. Our response to any change will vary depending on our genetic individuality. Our ability to adapt to changes that we make in our activity and environment can also vary from person to person.

Finally, the environments in which we find ourselves can be a major determinant of what we are exposed to, what we have available to us, and our ability to make changes.

We previously discussed the social challenges of location, association, cooperation, commitment, and cost. These are real and practical barriers that must be dealt with when it comes to executing a successful plan. Likewise, aspiration, inspiration, motivation, dedication, and cost have been discussed as challenges at the inner or psychological level.

The Concept of Energy. Scientists are still trying to fully understand energy, but it is really what drives us. Our efforts at enhancing our health are on one level an attempt to improve our energy. A detailed discussion of all of these concepts is beyond the scope of this book; however, we can easily understand the effects of physical energy. I often see patients in my practice who complain of having no energy. This, of course, is not literally true, but feeling a lack of physical energy can be a clue to a problem.

At the level of our social sphere, there is also a perceptible "collaborative energy" that takes place when we work with others toward a common goal. Think of the team spirit that is generated at a pep rally.

We can also experience a "spiritual energy." Although the hardest to understand, most cultures and individuals have an intuition that there exists more than that which we can experience with our five senses, and we feel a need to connect with that "spirit" at a fundamental level.

Although we do not live in an ideal world, our aim is to try to create as ideal a profile as possible, one in which our physical factors, while not perfect, exist within an acceptable range, our social supports are adequate to help us achieve these goals, and we understand our strengths and weaknesses enough to support the entire endeavor.

Optimal Health Profile

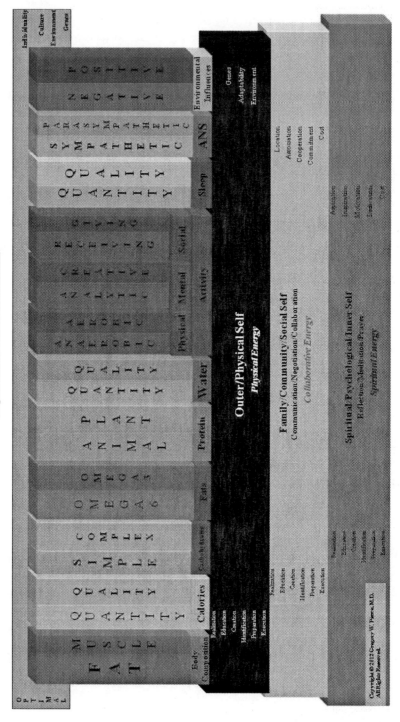

CHAPTER 9

Getting Started

This all looks nice on paper, but how practical is it? Why am I more likely to improve with this method compared to other approaches? The main difference with the *Building Health, Building Wellness* system is that there is no "system." I truly believe that with the proper information, you are perfectly capable of determining where you are and what steps are practical for you to employ or improve at any given point in time. Once you have decided what it is that you need to do, such as decreasing refined carbohydrates in your diet or increasing the omega-3 fats in your diet, you can read any of the many publications that speak to these issues.

Think of it as putting together a wardrobe. Most of us do not have the luxury of having all of our clothes tailor-made for us, but neither do we get all of our clothes from one place. We shop at different stores, putting together the clothes that are a good fit for us. We also wear different clothes at different times, and we often find that clothes that are a good fit for us are a poor fit for someone else.

Likewise, you may read several books that discuss "diet" or "exercise" and find that some of the concepts or advice may be a good fit for you and others may not. I don't think that you will find anyone else's approach a perfect fit for you, but you will be able to find some ideas that are good for you. If you want to find the program that is perfect for you, go to your local bookstore or library and find the book that has your picture on the front!

If you don't know where to start, here are a few ideas you can use that require no money and little effort.

Change how you eat

Do you really need a lesson in how to eat? Well, perhaps not a lesson, but your eating style can have subtle but significant influences on your health. For example, we all have heard that you should chew your food thirty-two times before swallowing. The exact number is not important, but the idea is a sound one. Outside of the particulars involved in the preparation of food, the mechanics of digestion begin with chewing. The purpose of chewing is to begin the process of breaking food down to allow it to be absorbed into our system. This is done through the mechanical action of chewing as well as through the action of mixing the food with saliva that contains enzymes that begin the digestive process. When we eat quickly and gulp our food, we bypass this important part of digestion.

Chewing food thoroughly also forces us to slow down as we eat. If you want to try a simple experiment, simply try to take twenty minutes to eat your meal. Believe me—it is not as easy as it sounds. When I first tried it, I found myself having to chew very slowly just to make the food last for the full twenty minutes. I also found myself actually tasting the food more than usual because I was taking my time. I noticed subtle distinctions in the flavor and texture of the food that I had not noticed before. I also noticed that at the end of the twenty minutes that I wasn't full, but I was totally satisfied, and there was still food left on my plate! I actually found that I had lost weight after a week of forcing myself to eat slowly. Perhaps one bad thing about fast food is that it is food fast! Eating slowly also leaves more time for conversation and further enjoyment of the meal. We go from eating food to enjoying a meal.

Most of us also benefit from being "grazers" rather than "gulpers." Eating small amounts frequently may serve us better than eating large amounts less frequently. The timing of meals may also be important for you. Eating your largest meal of the day at lunchtime may be good if you have a job that is physically demanding, but it may cause you to become very tired if you have a more sedentary job. Some people are used to a large breakfast; others are not. You should find a meal pattern that works the best for you. Because of our hurried and harried lifestyles, we may not be able to sit down to three well-spaced, nicely designed, and properly prepared meals every day. Try to get an idea of what your ideal pattern is, and strive toward it.

In addition, consider why you eat. Are you eating because it is time to eat, because you are hungry, because you are bored, because you are anxious or depressed, because you are at a social function, or for nutrition? There may be other reasons that you eat at any given time. Thinking about the reason for eating may help you to make better choices of what to eat and how much to eat.

Change your activity level

Again, I try to avoid using the word "exercise." We are all active to a certain extent, so it may make more sense and be easier for you to start by trying to simply increase the intensity or duration of the activities that you already perform. You are probably aware of and may employ many of these methods yourself, such as parking farther away in the parking lot, taking the stairs rather than the elevator, or taking a walk after dinner. You can probably think of several situations that you frequently encounter in which you can perform some extra physical activity. These are simple ways in which to get started.

Change how you think

Although we live in a competitive society and we are taught to be the best, many of us translate this into never being good enough. No matter how good we are, there is always someone better. Sometimes we slip into complacency: where I am is good enough; why rock the boat?

I believe that we must all start by accepting ourselves where we are and how we are. If we can't do that, we won't be happy fifty pounds lighter or $100,000 richer. We should also think of ways in which to improve ourselves consistently and constantly. This is a task that never ends, but it also makes for an easy beginning. Anything that we do to improve our health and wellness is a step in the right direction. If we think of it that way, we can see our life as one of many successes, both large and small, instead of one of many failures. It's not a matter of trying to achieve perfection; rather, it is a process of moving from good to better to best.

Time Management

"I don't have time for any of this!" This statement is probably true for most of us. No matter how early we get up in the morning, no matter how late we stay up at night, no matter how hard we work during the day, there are always things left undone. And these are the things that we must do for work, family, and others. How do we make the time to pay attention to our own health and well-being? And why do it now? There will be plenty of time later.

It has been said that everyone has twenty-four hours in his or her day—no more, no less. It's what you do with it that counts. There are many excellent books on time management, and I do not plan to compete with them here. There are so many, not because they all work, but because they all fail. It may be difficult to find the one that works best for you.

What has been most useful to me has been to change the way in which I think about time. It's not a finite quantity that has to be allocated to different activities during the day until it is all used up; instead, I think of the things that I want to do each day in terms of proportion.

My life is fairly simple, so there are only three ways in which I might spend my time:

- Private Time: Things that I do for myself—eating, sleeping, exercising, etc.
- Personal Time: Things that I do with/for my family and friends.
- Public Time: Things that I do for others—work, church activities, etc.

Granted, this is an overly simplistic way of thinking about daily activities, but it's a good place to start.

Take time to consider if you are spending your time as you should in each of these types of activities. If not, how can you change things in order to spend more time where you need or want to spend it? Keep in mind that the time it takes to do an activity also includes the time that it takes to prepare for and recover from that activity. For example, when we have others prepare meals for us, we can spend the time that we would have spent preparing a meal socializing with friends and family.

Likewise, preparing a meal can become a shared activity, turning time that might be spent alone into time that is spent with others.

Remember that we all have private, personal, and public lives, and we must find ways to spend an adequate amount of time and energy in each of these areas in order to achieve and maintain the best of health and wellness.

CHAPTER 10

DO YOU!

Some people say that if you know better, you do better. I am not convinced that this is entirely true. Knowledge is the basis for improvement, but it does not guarantee it.

Knowledge is the first step toward improvement, but not the final one. Self-knowledge is the real goal. What motivates me? What makes me happy? I will leave it to the professional philosophers and psychologists to struggle with these questions, but I will say something about happiness.

At some level, we all know (or think we know) what happiness is and what makes us happy. But is that all there is to it? I believe that we grow in terms of what happiness is and what makes us happy. Early in life we are made happy by "having," usually by having "things." Does anything make a child happier than a gift? As we mature, we learn to be happy by "doing." Initially doing for ourselves, such as when small children insist on feeding themselves, and then by doing for others. This continues as we get satisfaction from doing for our family and community and by doing things for ourselves, even when we're just keeping busy. As we continue to mature, we learn to be happy by just being. We may experience this sitting on the beach while on vacation, or we may observe this in older people who seem to be happy just sitting on the porch, watching the world go by.

Realizing that these are not separate and distinct stages and that there is considerable overlap and understanding what our "happiness ratio" is at any given time (i.e. how much happiness do we get from "having" vs. "doing" vs. "being") may help us to understand strategies that might be most helpful for us to enhance our health.

Master teacher Dr. Adolph Brown teaches: "Do you!" That is, measure where you are and what you need to do by your own yardstick, not that used by others. You are at a level of physical health unique to you; therefore, what it takes to improve and enhance your health will also be unique to you. Listen to what the experts have to say, but keep in mind that your aim is to determine how their advice applies to you. No book will apply to you one hundred percent, but you will find useful information in many of them. My father, Raymond O. Pierce, Jr., M.D. taught me: "Take your time and do it right." Doing it right means doing what is best for *you* right now.

CHAPTER 11

FINE TUNING:
TURNING FAILURE INTO SUCCESS

If at first you don't succeed, you're normal! The purpose of this book is not to tell you how to turn your imperfect life into one of perfection. Believe it or not, everyone leads an imperfect life. I think that we all know this, but we like to believe that "if I could only be like . . . ," "If only I had . . . ," or some other variation. We live in a culture of consumerism in which the job of the advertiser is to convince us that we have a problem then sell us a solution to that problem.

I will tell you this: where you are in your life right now is fine. Do you think that you are overweight? Well, you could weigh fifty pounds more than you do now, but you don't. Why not? You are obviously doing something right. In fact, you are probably doing many things correctly. So instead of looking at all of our shortcomings and trying to figure out how to fix them, why not look at the things that we are doing right and figure out how to enhance them?

We all know or have heard of people getting into a downward spiral, in which one thing goes wrong, then the next, and the next until their life is a total disaster. Why not start an upward spiral in which one thing goes right, then the next, and the next? Remember, it is not about perfection; it's about just doing better and being better today than yesterday. I'm sure that professional golfers wake up every morning and ask, "What can I do today to become a better golfer?" The answer is probably, "Not much!" Nevertheless, they still try to get just a little better. One more golf lesson for a professional golfer is likely to result in only a small improvement. But if I take one more golf lesson, I am likely to see a great deal of improvement because I have much more room for improvement.

If you have never done anything to improve your health, do not worry. If you are alive, you are at a beginning. You may have many ways in which you can improve, but who doesn't? I believe that the only thing that really matters is that we try to make progress. As we improve, our improvements become smaller and smaller, but they still come.

It also helps to understand how we really change. I do not believe that we improve in a linear fashion. I don't believe that you get twice as much improvement from walking two miles a day as you do from walking one mile a day. You might walk one mile a day—no change. Two miles a day—no change. Two and a half miles a day—suddenly, a big change. Three miles a day—no further change. You get the idea. We tend to change in thresholds or in a stair-step fashion. The problem is that we usually don't know how close to a threshold that we are. You might make a change and get a rapid improvement followed by continued effort with little or no change. Persistence results in eventually crossing another threshold, where we will again see results.

You may have heard the following story regarding one of the moon landings. An astronaut wanted to walk to the edge of a crater off in the distance. The problem on the moon is that there are no trees or buildings to give perspective, so by only looking, he could not judge how far away that the crater was. He started walking, keeping an eye on his watch. He had to return before he ran out of oxygen. After walking as long as he thought safe, he still had not reached his destination, so he turned around and came back. After he returned to Earth, calculations were done, and it was discovered that if he had walked for just one more minute, he would have reached his destination!

How often does this happen to us? We make a real effort toward change and see very little or no result. We give up and call ourselves a failure. Despite what we have been taught to believe, improvement is not what we measure on the scale or with blood tests or with a tape measure. Improvement begins once we make the decision to improve and take action. Studies have shown that people who make an effort to lose weight have improvements in their health even if they lose no weight at all! The idea is to think of ourselves as verbs (what we do) rather than nouns (what we are). When we improve what we do, we are improved. That does not mean that we shouldn't have specific goals or look at specific measurements, but they should be seen as guidelines, not necessarily goals.

It should be expected that, since we are not perfect, there will be good times and bad times, times when we do exactly as we should and times when we fail miserably. But overall, with time, we will improve as long as we continue to make an effort at changing.

Remember that wellness is a state of being—who we are and how we are at any given time—and health is a state of doing—what we are and where we are at any particular time. The goal is to work toward optimizing each of these parts of our lives.

CONCLUSION

A Life of Greatness

All of this might make interesting reading, but you have read many good books and still may not be where you want to be. You realize that reading words is not the same as taking action, so you take action. You have tried different approaches, listened to the tapes, gone to the support groups, joined the clubs, and bought the special foods, but you are right back where you started. You might rationalize that you are really not very bad off, and even if you led the perfect life and did everything just right, you still end up six feet under. So what's the point?

Well, I will leave that answer to the philosophers, but I will leave you with one last story. It is about Bob, an average person. He was assistant manager at a local bank, married with three children—two girls and a boy. He was troop leader for his son's Boy Scout troop and coached his daughters' junior soccer team. He was treasurer of the local Rotary club and on the deacon board at his church. He and his wife had lived long enough to witness the births of five grandchildren. By all accounts, Bob was a decent man who led a good life.

As it does for all of us, Bob came to the end of his days and found himself standing at the Pearly Gates talking to the chief angel.

"Welcome home, Bob. We have been waiting for you." But Bob didn't feel as joyous as he thought that he should, and this showed on his face. "What's wrong Bob?"

"Well," Bob replied, "on the way up here, I had the whole, 'life flashing before your eyes' thing and, well . . . I had a good life. No doubt about that. However, looking back, I think that I could have had a great life. Sure, I did okay for myself and my local community, but I think—no, I *know* I could have done better. Looking back, I get it now. I see many times when I could have done more and done better. I could have made a real difference in the world."

"Well, Bob, everyone feels that way, but you made it now. Come on in."

"No," Bob said, "I want to do it again. I want a do-over."

"What? Are you crazy?" the angel said. "We can't do that! If we let you go back, we would have to let everyone go back and live his or her life over again. Pretty soon, we wouldn't know who was coming or going. It would be a mess!"

"Come on," Bob pleaded. "You know that I could have really made the world a much better place. I could have brought much more happiness into the world."

After a pause, Bob got his answer. "Okay Bob, I've always liked you. Here's the deal. I can't let you go back and live your life all over again. It's just not done. But it's lunch time, and no one knows that you are here yet, so I can sneak you back for one minute."

"Only one minute?" Bob asked.

"Yes, one minute. You can choose which minute of your life to live over, but when you go back, you won't know that you are living that minute over again. It will be as though it was happening for the first time."

Dismayed, Bob replied, "I lived a very long life. One minute is not that long at all. What could I possibly do in one minute that would change my life from one of mediocrity to one of greatness that really improves the world?"

After another pause came the angel's final answer. "Perhaps you could make a decision."

Now, suppose that this was not a fictional story about a guy named Bob, but a story about *you*. Suppose you made the same deal that Bob made, and you got to choose one minute of your life to live over again. Suppose the minute that you chose to live over again was *this* minute right now, right here, reading these words. Suppose that you decided that *this* was the moment in which you could make a decision that would change your entire life. Change from an average life of contentment and mediocrity to a fantastic life of greatness, a most incredible life for you, your family, and the world.

I can't prove it, but perhaps you did make that deal, and this is the minute. What decision will you make—right now?

The world is waiting.

You only have one minute.

Common Stumbling Blocks and Building Blocks

Stumbling Blocks | Building Blocks

Stumbling Blocks	Building Blocks
I'm overweight, or I must go on a diet in order to be healthy.	I will improve my body composition.
Carbohydrates are bad for me.	I will consume the amount and type of carbohydrates best for me to improve my health.
Fat is bad for me.	I will consume the amount and type of fat that is best for me. I will also attain and/or maintain cholesterol levels that are appropriate for me.
I eat meat so I get plenty of the best protein, or I'm a vegetarian so I may not be getting enough protein.	I will consume the amount and type of protein that is best for me from good-quality sources.
I need to take vitamins and mineral supplements in order to be healthy.	I will make an effort to determine and consume the proper amount and types of vitamins and minerals that I need.
I drink plenty of water.	I will make sure that I get an adequate amount of water for me from the best sources, including food sources.

Stumbling Blocks	**Building Blocks**
I consume too many calories (I eat too much), or Calories in minus calories out determines my weight.	I will consume enough of the best quality calories for me. When I am hungry I will ask, "What am I hungry for?"
I must exercise in order to be healthy.	I will continue to improve the amount and type of activities that I engage in to promote my health and wellness.
I don't get enough sleep.	I will try to improve the quantity and quality of sleep that I get.
I'm too stressed out!	I will reduce the effects of stressors in my life by actively relaxing.
My success is entirely up to me, or My failure is entirely my own fault, or My family and friends are holding me back.	I will let my family and community become a part of my success.
Everything that I need for success is "out there."	Everything that I need for success is "in here."

About the Author

A native of Indianapolis, Indiana, Gregory W. Pierce, MD, is a Dean's List graduate of Wabash College in Crawfordsville, Indiana. He went on to earn a medical degree from Meharry Medical College in Nashville, Tennessee. While there, he served as president of his junior and senior classes and received several honors, including the Mosby Scholarship Book Award and the Upjohn Award for Excellence in Clinical and Academic Obstetrics and Gynecology, and induction into the Alpha Omega Alpha Honor Medical Society, which represents the top medical school graduates in the nation.

Upon completion of residency training in Family Medicine at the University of Tennessee, Dr. Pierce joined Family Health Associates, a private practice in Murfreesboro and Smyrna, Tennessee, where he practiced for six years.

Dr. Pierce subsequently moved to Virginia and joined Patient First as a full-time staff physician in Chesapeake and Virginia Beach. He also served as the Patient First Quality Assurance Committee's Primary Physician Inspector and as a member of the organization's continuing care committee before his appointment as Medical Director at the Patient First Indian River Road location. He served in that capacity until he accepted the position of Director of Continuing Education for Patient First.

Dr. Pierce is certified by the American Board of Family Medicine, and is a Fellow of the American Academy of Family Physicians.

He is the proud husband of Eurica Hill-Pierce, MD, and the proud father of two sons, Gregory and Matthew.

In addition to publishing, Dr. Pierce presents his ideas to audiences around the country. Drawing on his strong communication skills and over twenty years of practice experience as a family physician, Dr. Pierce specializes in discussing common and not-so-common topics relating to health and wellness in a unique way that helps his audiences to see these issues in an entirely new way.

Described by his audiences as "down to earth" and an "engaging speaker," Dr. Pierce leaves his audiences feeling educated, not exasperated. Presentations are tailor-made for the expected audience and include a variety of topics.

Dr. Piece's philosophy is that "there is always more to learn," and he is always looking for more to teach. His presentations are always updated with the latest in medical and scientific thought and always tempered by practicality, common sense, and humor. You may learn more or arrange for a live presentation of the concepts presented in this book at www.docandfriends.com.